FINDING DAD

PARANOID SCHIZOPHRENIA:
AN END TO THE SEARCH

AMANDA LAPERA

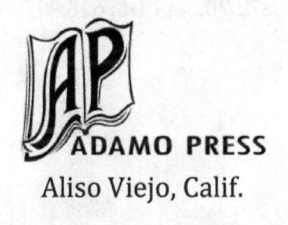

ADAMO PRESS
Aliso Viejo, Calif.

FINDING DAD, PARANOID SCHIZOPHRENIA:
AN END TO THE SEARCH

Copyright © 2024 by Amanda LaPera. All rights reserved.

Published by Adamo Press. Printed in the United States of America. No part of this book may be used or stored in any electronic form or reproduced in any manner whatsoever without prior written permission except in the case of brief quotations embodied in critical articles and reviews. For information, address: Adamo Press, 27068 La Paz Rd, Suite 102, Aliso Viejo, California 92656.

Adamo Press books may be purchased for educational, business, or sales promotional use. For information, email the Special Markets Department at info@adamopress.com.

Library of Congress Control Number: 2024948256

PUBLISHER'S CATALOGING-IN-PUBLICATION DATA

Names: LaPera, Amanda, 1978- author.

Title: Finding dad, paranoid schizophrenia: an end to the search / Amanda LaPera.

Description: Aliso Viejo, California: Adamo Press, [2024] | Includes bibliographical references. | Includes reading guide discussion questions.

Identifiers: ISBN: 978-0-9862471-6-3 (hardcover) | 978-0-9862471-7-0 (paperback) | 978-0-9862471-8-7 (eBook) | LCCN: 2024948256

Subjects: LCSH: LaPera, Amanda. | Paranoid schizophrenia. | Paranoid schizophrenics--Biography. | Paranoid schizophrenics--Family relationships. | Families of the mentally ill--Biography. | Children of the mentally ill--Biography. | Anosognosia--Patients--Biography. | Missing persons--Biography. | Mentally ill--Commitment and detention--Case studies. | BISAC: PSYCHOLOGY / Psychopathology / Schizophrenia. | BIOGRAPHY & AUTOBIOGRAPHY / Personal Memoirs. | HEALTH & FITNESS / Diseases & Conditions / Alzheimer's & Dementia.

Classification: LCC: RC514. L372 2024 | DDC: 616.89/8--dc23

10 9 8 7 6 5 4 3 2

Cover design by Fiona Jayde

www.adamopress.com

*Dedicated to those who haven't found their loved ones:
May you find peace*

CONTENTS

PART ONE: THE SEARCH (2017-2018)

Chapter 1: The Call 1
Chapter 2: Halva 7
Chapter 3: Return to Sender 10
Chapter 4: Affirmation 14
Chapter 5: Big News 20
Chapter 6: Found 25

PART TWO: CONNECTIONS (2019)

Chapter 7: Heart Attack 35
Chapter 8: Delayed 40
Chapter 9: Now Boarding 46
Chapter 10: Arrival 49
Chapter 11: Recognition 56
Chapter 12: The Prophet 58
Chapter 13: Vitals 62
Chapter 14: The Surrogate 68
Chapter 15: Meltdown 75
Chapter 16: The Fight 81
Chapter 17: NAMI 87
Chapter 18: The Nurse 93
Chapter 19: POA 96
Chapter 20: Deep-Dish Pizza 99
Chapter 21: Grandpa 101
Chapter 22: The Collaboration 109
Chapter 23: Fireworks 114
Chapter 24: Finding Dad 119
Chapter 25: Missing Money 125

Chapter 26: Things Overlooked..128
Chapter 27: Clothing 132
Chapter 28: Mounting Problems..135
Chapter 29: The Engagement..145
Chapter 30: The Missing Years..150
Chapter 31: Keep the Hope Alive 153
Chapter 32: The Shoes 157
Chapter 33: Getting Nowhere..160
Chapter 34: The Outing...163
Chapter 35: Gaining Access..168

PART THREE: COMPLICATIONS (2020-2021)

Chapter 36: Forensic Accounting 173
Chapter 37: Signs of Love 179
Chapter 38: In Limbo...181
Chapter 39: Normalcy 185
Chapter 40: New Prospects...189
Chapter 41: Dress Shopping 196
Chapter 42: Making Plans 198
Chapter 43: All That Glitters Isn't Gold 201
Chapter 44: 2-20-2020..204
Chapter 45: The Move...208
Chapter 46: The World Shuts Down..212
Chapter 47: Covid-19 217
Chapter 48: Belligerence...222
Chapter 49: Pneumonia 226
Chapter 50: The Plot 231
Chapter 51: The Distance Between 234
Chapter 52: Seeking Answers...239
Chapter 53: The Results 243
Chapter 54: The Return...247

Chapter 55: Ohio 252

Chapter 56: The Trek 254

Chapter 57: Accusations 259

Chapter 58: The Psych Ward 263

Chapter 59: Checkers and Chess 268

Chapter 60: The Speech Therapist 272

Chapter 61: Misunderstood 274

Chapter 62: "Are You There, Dad?" 279

Chapter 63: Sense of Urgency 283

PART FOUR: UNDERSTANDING (2022)

Chapter 64: Dysphagia 289

Chapter 65: Reassurances 292

Chapter 66: Perilous 297

Chapter 67: Making Peace 304

Chapter 68: Helpless 307

Chapter 69: Homeward Bound 310

Chapter 70: "I Love You" 314

AFTERWORD 319

OBITUARY 321

RESOURCES 322

AUTHOR'S STATEMENT 323

ACKNOWLEDGEMENTS 324

READING DISCUSSION QUESTIONS 325

ABOUT THE AUTHOR 327

FINDING DAD

PARANOID SCHIZOPHRENIA: AN END TO THE SEARCH

PART ONE

THE SEARCH (2017-2018)

CHAPTER ONE

The Call

DECEMBER 21, 2017, 5:47 PM
Orange County, California

I fumbled in my purse for my cell phone and checked the caller ID: It was the Orange County Sheriff's Department. Had they found Dad's body? I held the phone in my hand and let it ring again.

The woman on the other line announced herself as an officer from the Homicide and Missing Persons Department. I knew who she was.

"Just got off the phone with Homeland Security," she said. "They found your father."

"Dead?"

"No, alive."

My stomach fluttered. I sat down, lucky enough to find an open bench in the crowded mall with all the Christmas shoppers hurrying about. The carolers and snowflake décor faded into the distance.

After more than six years of communicating with the authorities, my hopes of finding Dad had dwindled. I expected to eventually to get *the call*, but *this* wasn't it.

"Alive?" I took a deep breath. "Where?"

Had he been arrested in Israel, again? Did the mafia get him?—all valid possibilities considering Dad's history. Immersed in delusions, Dad had traversed the globe as a self-proclaimed Prophet of God before he disappeared.

"He's in the US," she said.

I reached in my purse for a paper. I cradled the phone against my shoulder and uncapped a pen. "Where is he now?"

"They won't say."

"What? You're a cop. Shouldn't they have to tell you?"

"I've tried. All they're saying is they came in contact with him, advised him of his missing person status, he said he wasn't missing, and that's it. They asked him to call you."

Which of course he wouldn't do. "That's all you know?"

"They found him at a facility."

A lanky older woman with glasses perched on the end of a pronounced nose set down her shopping bags and took a seat beside me on the bench.

"Facility?" I lowered my voice. "What, the ER for another heart attack? Another mental hospital for another suicide attempt? Is he in Chicago?"

"I don't know. Honestly, Amanda, it's frustrating for me, too."

"What do we do next?"

"Nothing. They took him off the list."

I dropped the pen and paper on my lap and took the phone in my hand. "They can do that? What about the DNA samples?"

"They've been dumped from the database."

"Are you kidding? How are they going to identify Dad's body when…" The woman next to me raised an eyebrow, tucked a short gray curl behind her ear and leaned a little closer. I turned in the other direction, cupped my hand over my mouth, and continued. "When Dad is found dead on the streets, how will they contact me if he's off the missing persons list?"

"Technically, Joseph is no longer missing."

I sighed and closed my eyes. "Can't exactly say he's been found." I softened my tone. "Thanks. I know you've tried, but I guess this is it."

"You can reach out to me to file another report if you locate him and he disappears again."

"Sure."

I zoned out while she, a stranger I'd only met in person once, offered words of comfort. I didn't need comfort. I needed answers.

After I hung up, I sat in stunned silence. I'd assumed Dad was dead, but he was alive and gone, again. This cat and mouse game was getting old.

I'd spent a decade searching for Dad. And now, the authorities wouldn't share his location—a painful reminder of how medical professionals had hidden behind HIPAA in a misguided attempt to protect his privacy. They withheld info that would've helped us to help him. Hence why, after he developed late-onset Paranoid Schizophrenia and grandiose delusions at fifty-three, Dad ended up on the streets. We found out that sometimes nobody shares information to help a family track down a loved one with a severe mental illness as long as they're alive. The cruel irony.

In no mood to buy gifts, I headed home.

I pulled my "Dad" file out from the filing cabinet and brought it to my desk. I jotted down the date, time, and information gathered earlier. Then I conference-called my stepmom, Hilda, my older sister Jackie, and younger brother Keith. We were the only immediate family members of Dad's who were still alive.

With everyone on the call, I couldn't help but wondering if things would have turned out differently if we all had communicated this much when Dad first got sick in 1996.

I delivered the unexpected update.

"Oh, praise the Lord. What can we do, my, Amandy?" Hilda asked, in her Argentinian accent.

"I don't even know where to start," I said.

"What are our options?" Keith asked—always the practical one.

"I can't file another missing person's report unless he shows back up in California then disappears again and—"

"How likely is that?" Jackie's voice quivered. "He doesn't know where I live, right, Amanda? Because I told you not to give him my address—"

"No, he only knows mine. But he wasn't exactly happy with me the last time we talked."

"Why is that, Amandy? Your daddy wouldn't be mad at you."

"Remember how he reacted to my book?" During my last phone call with Dad, I told him about my book, *Losing Dad, Paranoid Schizophrenia: A Family's Search for Hope*. I should've known better. With his anosognosia—

an inability to understand he was sick, which is typical of those suffering from paranoid schizophrenia—he had little to no insight into his mental illness. The moment I said the word "psychology," I was from the devil, like my stepmom, and dead to him.

It had hurt me to hear the accusations of betrayal in Dad's silence. His little girl, the one he'd always asked to navigate the fold-out maps for him during our road trips, no longer an ally in his eyes.

After that, I cut ties with my literary agent, especially because she envisioned my book to be a worldwide-adventures-with-crazy-dad type of story. But from the beginning, I intended to tell our family's story, the story of how mental illness affects everyone—spouse, children, parents, coworkers, and community. I wasn't looking for an incredible journey down the vortex of Dad's insanity, but more a case study, the kind that shows the hidden and painful reality lived by too many families.

"Yeah, that was stupid," Keith said. "Why did you tell him? It's not like he would've figured it out."

"Dad was always a private person," Jackie said. "I don't disagree with her advice. It was a good idea to tell him you were putting his picture on the cover. He had a right to know."

"He may not even remember the book," Keith said. "Where do you think he is?"

"If I had to guess," I said, "probably Chicago."

"Why?" Keith asked. "His parents are dead. He's an only child. Not like he talks to anyone else in the family. Pretty much burned those bridges."

"Did you call Dad's cousin?" Jackie asked. "Maybe she knows."

"No." I sighed. "I haven't talked to her since we planned Grandma's funeral—"

"Because Dad wasn't around to help," Jackie said. "This whole thing is bullshit."

"*Ai-yi-yi,*" Hilda said. "Your poor daddy. He was a great man, a great husband. I'm sorry for you kids." She sniffled. "And he left me here all alone. If I could sell this stupid house…"

A disturbing thought flashed in my mind—the ominous phone call Hilda had received years earlier from a stranger.

"What if someone's taking advantage of Dad?" I asked.

"Oh, no, Amandy. That man." Hilda paused. "You need to find your daddy."

Back on November 11, 2013 at 8 PM, I'd received a panicked call from Hilda. A mysterious man in his fifties or sixties had phoned her house in West Virginia. In a whisper, he had warned Hilda that Dad was in danger.

At first, she thought it a prank. But the stranger knew Dad's full name, her full name, the names of all three of Dad's kids, his birthdate, his social security number. He knew Dad was receiving income from three sources, including a pension, his social security, and probably something else.

Hilda knew this was true, because she was getting the other half of Dad's pension and social security checks, something she and Dad arranged shortly after he abandoned her.

The man continued, speaking in a low voice, "He's living in a house. I think these people are taking advantage of him."

Hilda pushed for details: Who, where, when, how?

"Someone's coming. I have to go." The line disconnected.

The next day, Hilda went in person to the social security office and reported the call. She spoke to the police department to figure out how to report potential elder abuse, but hit a wall at every attempt because she didn't have the phone number—Hilda didn't have caller ID—and we didn't have enough details.

Yep. Mental illness sucks.

Because of Hilda's insistence, I assured her I would try to track him down. I did an internet search for all hospitals with emergency rooms and all mental hospitals in the Chicago area. Then, one-by-one, I phoned: Masonic Medical Center, University of Illinois Hospital, Kindred Hospital, Swedish Covenant Hospital, Mercy Hospital, Northwestern Memorial Hospital, Cook County Hospital on Harrison, Provident Hospital of Cook County, Chicago Lakeshore Hospital and their psychiatric hospital, Methodist Hospital, Thorek Memorial Hospital, Weiss Memorial Hospital, and St. Joseph's Hospital—where Dad had two heart surgeries, one in November 2004 and the other in April 2005.

Each time, I asked to speak to Dad who I identified as a patient at their facility. No matter who I called, I got the same response, "I'm sorry, there's no patient here by that name."

I phoned them back to ask if my dad had been admitted and released. At this request, suspicions were raised and I got a lot of, "We can't share that information with you."

So, I gave up.

Maybe I was wrong. Perhaps Dad wasn't in Chicago. But it wasn't possible to call every hospital in every state. I'd been through all this drama with Dad before. I couldn't do it again. I had other things to worry about in my life now—my two sons, a new relationship (My first husband and I divorced back in 2013—one of my better decisions), and my cervical spinal stenosis which was causing increasing amounts of neck pain.

After these dead ends, I accepted the new reality—Dad was missing. Again.

So, I went on with my life. Besides which, I'd mourned his death too many times to count. The sting was lessening each time. That or I'd become numb.

CHAPTER TWO

HALVA

I BOLTED UPRIGHT and wiped my eyes, the dream still vivid. The memory, as clear as the day it happened decades earlier, played out in my mind while I lay there in bed.

I was twelve. My arms were crossed as I sat back in the red checkered chair at the kitchen table, playing blackjack with Dad. On the table were stacks of plastic red, white, and blue gambling chips. It was nearing midnight and the house was quiet—only the two of us still awake.

"Well, why can't I?" I said, pointing to the six of hearts and the six of spades in front of me.

Dad took off his wire-framed glasses to wipe the bridge of his nose, only a shade darker than the rest of the fair skin he'd inherited from his Ashkenazi Jewish ancestry. He rubbed a hand over his thinning brown hair and stared at me with his pale blue eyes.

He slid a paper over to me. "See? The dealer has a seven. If he has a ten, he stands. You don't want to split on a six."

"But you said I could split on doubles."

"Technically, yes." He pointed to his handwritten notes and the Hoyle's Rules of Games book. "Look at the odds. Best not to split, unless you have eights."

"I give up. Let's play something else. How about chess?"

"Patience. You'll get it." He opened up a box of See's Candies and slid it over to me. "Here."

I pulled a piece out, nibbled on a corner and let the chocolate melt in my mouth. I took another tiny taste and closed my eyes to focus on the flavor like Dad always did.

I opened my eyes and tapped two fingers on the table. "Hit."

He flipped a nine. Twenty-one.

"What does the dealer have?"

Dad flipped over the dealer's second card. "A king. Dealer holds at seventeen."

While Dad stacked up my winning chips, I asked, "Can I see the next couple?"

He showed me the cards. If I had split, I would've had a six and a nine, then a face card. Twenty-five. Would've busted. My other hand? He flipped a face card. A six and a ten. Sixteen. Would've lost to the dealer's seventeen. Dad, as usual, was right.

He shuffled the cards and packed them away. "Time for bed, Amanda."

I pushed in my chair and gave him a kiss on the cheek. "I love you."

He hugged me. "I love you, too."

I squeezed my eyes shut tight. These dreams and memories of Dad were becoming frequent again. The father I grew up with was gone. I'd long accepted that. I moved on. So why was I still thinking of the past?

Spring 2018. A pleasantly warm and sunny Southern California day, the kind that inspires hikes along tree-covered trails or kayaking. Instead, I tidied up the house and checked off the to-do list of chores. Super exciting.

My boyfriend Leo, whom I'd been dating since the summer of 2015, came home and set groceries on the counter. My friends referred to him as the "unicorn" on account of his many talents—cooking, dancing, singing, fixing anything around the house, and more.

"I got something for you," he said. "Something sweet."

Never a bad time for chocolate in my world.

He pulled out a box of confections and handed it to me.

Halva. Oh my God—*Halva*.

I dropped it and ran to my room crying.

"Damn it," he said from the other room. "Something told me not to get it. I think you said your dad got it for you."

Yeah. I guess I wasn't over the dad thing as much as I thought. That or I was repressing my worries and fears because of my impotence to do anything about it.

Leo didn't buy me Halva again and the memories of Dad faded away. Hopefully my father was getting whatever medical attention he needed, wherever he was.

CHAPTER THREE

Return to Sender

On Father's Day, 2018, six months after the jarring call from the sheriff's department, I mailed Dad a card same as I did most years. I sent it to his PO Box in Chicago, which felt like sending something into the black void of the universe. Unlike my lengthy letters in the past, I only wrote "I love you and miss you" and signed my name. I added a couple of stick figures to represent the two of us, some hearts, X's and O's, then dropped it in the mail and forgot about it.

Summer break couldn't come soon enough. As a high school English teacher, I felt satisfied but emotionally and mentally drained from another year with over a hundred and fifty teenagers who couldn't wait to get out of there.

My sons Justin, now twenty-one and working a full-time job, and David, on the verge of eleven and the cusp of middle school, both usually participated in annual road trips with me, a tradition I carried on from my childhood with Dad.

I remembered the longest road trip I took with my dad when he drove us—me, Hilda, and Keith, Jackie was already away in college—north from Southern California, through Oregon to Washington, where we'd take a ferry boat across the strait to the city of Victoria on the island of Vancouver, Canada.

It was the summer of 1992. While we waited in a tourist store on the Olympic Peninsula for our scheduled loading time, I browsed the shelves of Troll dolls with their rainbow assortment of bright hair and varied outfits. Rather than discourage me from such trivial keepsakes, Dad approached me with a grin on his face. From behind his back, he produced a troll with bright blue hair and a blue and white outfit emblazoned with the Star of David, even though neither he, as a single child, nor his parents, had ever been religious.

"Can I?" I asked, with two other dolls in my hands.

Dad nodded and bought me all three, which kept me busy until it was time to return to the ferry station.

He wasn't fond of heights or the beach or traveling on the ocean, but he managed to keep his meal down during the short trip while I gazed out the window at the rolling waves. I watched as we parted a path through the water, creating a wake to follow behind.

Once on the island, after a Mr. Belvedere look-alike checked us into our hotel, Dad had us on our way to visit Butchart Gardens. Hilda loved roses and gardening and he loved nature as did I. The line of cars moved at a snail's pace. At least we could see the sign.

"Dad," I said. "Why is it called butt chart?"

He chuckled. "It's not. It's pronounced Butchart."

"But it's spelled butt chart."

"No, it's not."

"Well, I'm going to call it butt chart anyways."

Dad shook his head, held his finger to his lips for me to shush, and pointed out the window. He spoke softly, "Just look with your eyes."

Whilst in nature, he always encouraged us to quiet down and observe with our eyes, so as to absorb our surroundings. That's how I came to value the ridges on the barks of the Giant Sequoias and Redwoods, and the individual veins on each leaf of forest trees.

I recreated this road trip with my own boys. In the summer of 2013, I drove Justin and David up to the west coast and crossed into Canada where we had High Tea at the Rose Garden in Butchart Gardens.

Time to plan another trip. I spread out paper maps across the carpet. I opened the AAA TourBook and highlighted various things to do and see, and yelled out for David and Justin to come in the room and join me. David sat cross-legged on the floor and flipped through the guidebook without much enthusiasm.

Justin leaned against the doorframe. "I'm not going."

"What? Why?" I asked.

"I can't get time off work."

"But we always go together."

"I have a job now. I can't go."

David stared up at me and shrugged his shoulders.

"I can't do all that driving by myself," I said. "It would only be me and David."

"Don't look at me," David said. "I can't drive."

So, our plans changed. Instead of pulling several days of ten-hour drives by myself, I planned to take David along with me on short last-minute trip to Cabo San Lucas, Mexico with some friends.

While I browsed for airline tickets, my dogs barked as the mailman approached. I shushed them and opened the mailbox to find a blue envelope that had seen better days. I turned it over and paused. It was a card I had sent to Dad. It had been labeled "**RETURN TO SENDER, NO SUCH STREET, UNABLE TO FORWARD**" with the date of June 1, 2018. In the ten years of mailing him birthday cards and holiday letters, this had never happened.

Wait. The envelope I sent last week was white; this one was blue. Dad's address was there. Was his P.O. Box full? Hadn't he checked it? Then I saw the postmark—June 17, 2017. I had sent the card a year ago. Whatever this meant, in the pit of my stomach it didn't feel right.

Back when Dad and I still spoke, before he disappeared the last time, he told me he prepaid his Chicago P.O. Box as far in advance as they'd let him. Ever since then, this had been my one-sided communication with him.

The yellow strip on the bottom of the envelope indicated the mail was undeliverable. I flashed back to the call from the OC sheriff six months prior. Was there a connection? Even if there was, what could I legally do?

The last time I phoned the Chicago post office, a decade earlier, they had been less than helpful.

Laurie's name popped into my head, Dad's cousin, the one who helped my grandparents to set up a special trust for Dad. She and her husband owned a law firm in the suburbs, not far from Chicago. I called her office, but no one answered. I left a message then tried her cell.

"Amanda?" Laurie sounded surprised, probably because we hadn't spoken in years. "What's wrong?"

"The Post Office returned mail I sent to Dad. His P.O. Box is closed."

She was quiet for a moment. "Well, that's not good."

I relayed the update I had received from the Orange County Sheriff's Department last December.

"Where do you think he is?" she asked.

"I have no idea. But I need to find out. Can you help?"

"Have you called Melody at the trust company?"

"Would she be willing to share information with me?"

"I'll give her a call." She paused. "I hope you find him."

I waited.

The next day, I got a text from Laurie: Go ahead and call Melody

It was after three o'clock in California which meant five o'clock Central time. I'd have to wait until the next day.

The following morning, I dialed her number.

Melody answered right away. "I was expecting your call."

CHAPTER FOUR

AFFIRMATION

I BRUSHED my fingers along the blue envelope on the table next to me. "I'm concerned about Dad," I said. "I got mail returned."

"So did we," Melody said. "We're worried, too."

"Have you seen him lately?"

"Not in a long time, nearly two years ago. We'd been transferring small monthly distributions to his bank account but paused that last year when we were unable to make contact with him."

"Dad never had a cell phone. As far as I know, he hasn't had an apartment or a place to stay. How were you talking to him before?"

"He checked in every so often. He seemed to enjoy stopping by and visiting with us."

I felt envious that he visited the bank but not me. Is it because I didn't let him drain money from me or his parents while they were alive? I told Melody about the National Missing Persons Database and updated her on his technically "found" but in reality, still missing status.

"I didn't know all that," she said. "We ran a skip trace on him."

"Did you find anything?" Before I became a teacher, I worked for a finance company as a credit manager. I knew about collections and skip tracing even though I hadn't personally done one. Creditors run reports to locate people who default on debt by tracing every address used on public records. This would include official documents, credit applications, and more. In his case, I knew it wouldn't have pulled up any credit cards or loans—Dad didn't believe in all that and, with his paranoia, had reverted to only paying in cash.

"Yes. We got back several addresses, including a Holiday Inn where he'd stayed in the past, but he hasn't been there in a while. So, there are three recent addresses in particular that we focused on—a homeless shelter, a medical facility, and a hospital—all in Chicago."

"Did you get a hold of him?"

"We tried. Because we aren't next of kin, nobody will share information with us. I actually had it on my list to call you."

"I thought you couldn't give me any details about him."

"We're in a tough situation. We have a fiduciary duty to take care of him, but we're now at a spot where we can't do that without your help." She gave the phone numbers.

Again, the irony. *You can't help me find my dad to help him, until it's too late for me to help him.*

"I'll let you know if I find him." I doubted I would have any luck.

Unfortunately, I didn't know which addresses were used when. If he had been spotted in a facility in December, it could've been either the hospital or the other medical facility.

Multiple scenarios played out in my mind. Maybe he'd been in the facility, then hospitalized, then taken refuge in a shelter, and was alive. Or he was at a shelter, then the hospital, then the facility, and was possibly still alive. Or maybe he was in the shelter, then the facility, then the hospital, then died. I hoped it wasn't the latter.

I called the hospital, but as expected, I got zero information from them. I figured they wouldn't tell me if he'd been admitted or for what without a court order or Power of Attorney form, neither of which I had.

I phoned the medical facility.

"I'm looking for information on one of your patients," I said, "Joseph—"

"I'm sorry," the receptionist said, "but I'm unable to verify any resident by that name."

Resident? What kind of facility was this one? "So, he's there?"

"I didn't say that."

"So, he's not there?"

"I didn't say that, either. Who is this?"

"His daughter." I tried to explain my dad's homeless background, but she cut me off.

"Ma'am, I can't give you any information."

I hung up and paced the room. Maybe he was there. Maybe not. Now I felt more compelled to get answers. I dialed the homeless shelter's number.

"Can I speak with someone there about a person named Joseph staying there? It's his daughter."

"Sorry but that's private information. We can't share anything." They hung up.

So, that's another maybe. I figured I'd wait until after my trip to Mexico to try again. Then I'd try again and again and again until somebody told me something. Maybe they would if I annoyed the hell out of them.

After we landed at the airport in Cabo San Lucas, I can't say I was disappointed when I realized David and I didn't have cell coverage. Perhaps that was the only reason I was able to disconnect from the emotional drama of Dad for a few days. Focusing on snorkeling, boat trips, and zip lines kept my mind busy.

But as soon as I unpacked my bags at home, the returned envelope and the possible leads resumed their front position in my mind. So, the next morning, I phoned the shelter and asked to speak with the manager. I got his voicemail and left a message.

I researched the medical facility that popped up when I searched for the phone number; it seemed to be a skilled nursing rehabilitation center with some long-term care beds. I called again but didn't say anything about Dad. Instead, I asked for the name and extension of the director. They gave me the information and transferred me to a voicemail but I didn't leave a message.

I reached out to Melody. "Nothing yet. If I can confirm where he is, I'll let you know."

"And I'll do the same," she said.

After a couple hours, I tried the shelter again and asked for the manager by name. This time, I got through.

"Before you hang up, my dad has been missing for over ten years and has untreated paranoid schizophrenia. Please help me find him. We want to bring him home and get him help."

The manager declined to give me information and told me to talk to the police.

"The police won't help us. I had him in the Database of Missing Persons and they still refused to help. Do you know he has three kids and four grandkids out in California looking for him? He has a wife who searched for him on the streets of Chicago in the snow. She couldn't find him. The police didn't help her. Now she's stuck by herself in West Virginia. My dad's parents are dead. Please, please, can you at least tell me if you've seen him? Ever? Please."

He gave a long pause. "Yes, I do know your dad. He stayed here a while. Nice guy, but the mental illness thing explains a lot."

"He was there. But he's not there anymore?"

"No."

"Did he just walk out and leave? Did something happen to him? Did he die?"

"I don't know. All I can tell you is that he left here in an ambulance."

"When? Was it another heart attack or did he try to hurt himself? Hurt someone else?"

"I can't give you any more information."

I thanked him again and documented the information in a notebook. Before I could call the long-term care place back, I took a deep breath. Even if I could get more information, if they said he left before or after the shelter, the news wouldn't be good.

It took several attempts over the next few days before I was finally able to get the facility director on the line. I went through the same script with her.

"Look I'm sure you know this," she said, "but I can't share any information with you."

"The homeless shelter at least told me something. Please."

"I can't."

"I don't know what else to do." Then an idea popped in my head. "Do you have access to the Internet?"

"Yes, why?"

"Please Google 'Losing Dad' and my name, Amanda." I knew what she'd find. My book. "Is the man on the cover of that book currently in your facility?"

I heard the slightest gasp on the other end. Affirmation.

"I'm Amanda. That's my dad." I closed my eyes. Dad was alive. I found him. I pondered… How much information could I get from her without pushing too far? Play it casual.

"I'm sure you've heard plenty of stories from a lot of your patients," I said. "But everything he's told you is probably real. He traveled as a self-proclaimed prophet-of-God to over thirty countries. He came back to America and disappeared, homeless, living on the streets. But he's got a Master's Degree. He's brilliant."

"Wow. I mean we don't believe everything we hear… I should read your book."

She was a reader! Entice her, carefully. "I can send you a copy. He's been in the Missing Persons database for over ten years. Do you know he's married with three kids, and has grandkids he's never met? The whole thing is unbelievable, which is why I wrote the book. It won a national book award in psychology. I do speaking engagements to tell our family's story."

"Incredible. And you've been looking for him this entire time? Most patients end up here because they don't have families or they've been cut off. Most don't get visitors."

"We're all out here in California. I would absolutely come visit him, but I don't want to scare him away—he might end up back out on the streets. That's my nightmare—Dad dying on the streets alone, with no one even able to identify his body. I don't want to lose him again. He'd refused treatment for a long time."

"He's accepting treatment here," she said. "Sorry I just looked at the clock. I need to get going."

"You have no idea how much this means to me and my family to have found him."

Unbelievable. I sat there and stared at the wall. Could I be sure it was really him? No, not until I could stare into his eyes in person. That's the only way to confirm I'd really found him. Or at least that's when my heart would believe it.

I had gotten so used to it all, to finding him then losing him, that I really didn't allow myself to feel relief or to feel anything at all. Avoid emotions to avoid pain and hurt and disappointment—this was a lesson I'd been taught by the universe repeatedly.

I had found him. Maybe. But I didn't want to lose him. With the precariousness of the situation, I needed a strategy. I would try to build a relationship with the director then attempt to enlist her help to regain Dad's trust. But first, I would tell my family.

CHAPTER FIVE

Big News

Days passed and I staved off emotions that threatened to flood through me after the initial shock wore off. I was so used to going into business mode—setting goals and accomplishing them. Complete the checklist. Make the calls. Keep my emotions on the back burner.

But even after so many years mourning his loss, after the tears and anger and frustration, despite my fervent denials, I realized a strong feeling was still there—love.

Love is the only reason I kept up this frustrating search for a dad who no longer existed. Why? Because the dad I grew up with didn't deserve to die alone on the streets.

I decided not to tell Melody at the trust company yet. There were a couple of reasons for that. One, what if it wasn't really him? I wanted to personally confirm before saying anything. And, two, what if they got to him first, helped him relocate and he disappeared again? Then he could end up back on the streets and we'd all be no better off. After I could make in-person contact with him to confirm he was alive, then I'd let Melody know.

But contacting Dad was tricky. I'd spoken with the director at the facility a few more times as well as a few of their social workers. Together we came up with a plan: I'd send Dad a box of See's chocolates—his favorite—but wouldn't reach out to him yet. See how he reacted.

It was the week of Dad's 75th birthday, July 2018. I phoned Hilda first.

"What is new with my Amandy?" Hilda said. "I was going to call you. I have news for you. You wouldn't believe it."

"What?" Did she already know? Had they contacted her?

"I finally sold this stupid house. It's been so many years. Your daddy paid too much for this place and it's been so hard. I'm too tired of this, so now it's finally done."

"Sold the house? Where are you going?"

"That's what I want to tell you. I'm moving back to Argentina."

"Argentina? Why? Why not come back out to California where we all are?"

She sighed. "I'm so sorry, dear. I can't. My sister and all my family are there."

Weren't we her family, too? "This just happened?"

"Yes. You know I've been trying for years to sell this stupid house. Someone comes to buy, then no, they change their mind. Finally, finally, I sold it."

"Hilda." This was hard for me to process too much at once. "I think I found Dad."

"What? Where?"

"Chicago."

"Oh, Amandy. Thank the Lord! You couldn't believe how much I prayed for him. Is Daddy okay?"

"I think so, but I haven't talked to him yet."

"But he is okay? I pray to the Lord he is okay. I waited so long for him."

"I know." I've always felt she had the strength of Penelope. "Why have you never moved on? Have you never wanted to date anyone else?"

"Oh, no. Why? Why would I do that? I love him … he is the only person for me. Despite all those stupid women, I couldn't handle that, you know that, Amandy, but still … it's so sad. So many years …. Maybe he wants to come down to Argentina … to come live with me? Maybe you could ask him? We could stay down by the beach house. He always liked it down there. Oh, that would be so wonderful."

I hated to destroy her hope, but her wishes could not become reality. Considering his last chilly reception towards my stepmom, his wife, I doubted that even if he could leave Chicago, that he would.

"I don't think so," I said. "He's in a facility."

"Facility? What kind of facility?"

"A nursing home I think." I cringed telling her this.

"Oh." She was quiet for a moment. "That's so sad. I'm so sorry to hear that. Well, I don't know what to do. I already sold the house. I have my ticket to Argentina. Thank God for my friends here who've helped me."

"No, you go. We'll figure it out."

"Are you sure? I could go to be with him if he wanted me to."

I couldn't let her stay trapped here any longer. Hilda had been in limbo for over eighteen years. I couldn't understand how she had faithfully waited that long believing against all odds that her husband would return. It simply wasn't fair to her. She needed permission to live her life, to move on.

"No," I said, "don't stay for Dad. Go be with your family, but it would be nice if we could see you soon, too. I know Jackie really misses you a lot."

"I know. I know. It's hard for me though. I can't explain it. It's very hard. Just so many things with your Daddy and you kids reminds me of him. It's not easy for me. But I love you all. Promise me, you will tell me how he is. I will pray for him."

After speaking with Hilda, I told Jackie that Hilda had sold the house.

"When was she going to tell us?" Jackie said. "Why not come here?"

"Who's going to help her?" I said. "Down there she has her family."

"We are her family."

"In brighter news, I think I found Dad."

It was a lot to process for all of us: Hilda leaving for Argentina, finding Dad. The irony of the timing was not lost on me. Hilda had been married to Dad for more than thirty years, half of which were spent in his absence after his illness hit. Every time I spoke with Hilda for the past eighteen years, she'd ask me if I'd heard from him, always worried if he'd ever be found and if he was okay, or even alive. And now, it was too late for her to ever get him back.

I told Keith the bombshell news about finding Dad and Hilda leaving.

"Do you blame her?" he said. "She's waited too long as it is. At least now she knows."

"Yeah, I'm sure it's better than not knowing," I said. "I want to send Dad chocolate."

"Let me know how much it costs, and I'll send you half," Keith said.

I didn't question why, especially knowing that Keith, because of the past, was the least likely person to connect with Dad if given the chance. After all, he was only a teenager when Dad lost his mind, accused Keith of plotting against him, and kicked him out of the house. Understandably, Keith had been the quickest one out of the three of us siblings to close the chapter on our former father and move on. So, whenever he offered anything towards Dad in any way, I appreciated his emotional generosity.

To continue to build a relationship with the staff, Keith and I sent two boxes with clear instructions that one was for the staff and the other was for Dad.

I checked back in a week later.

"Yes, he enjoyed it," a staff member said. "He finished the whole box."

"He didn't ask about me, or who sent it?"

"No. Most of the patients here don't get visitors or calls. Your dad has never had any. To be honest, we figured he didn't have any living relatives. I'm glad for him that you're trying."

By the fall, the director had quit her job and was replaced. Social workers came and went. So did nurses. There was high turnover there. Each time, I made an effort to connect with the new person, explain the situation, and stay in contact, to ask about Dad without pressing for details or information that would cause pushback.

With each new person, it became the norm that Joseph's daughter was involved in his care and to share limited information with me as if it had always been the case. They said my dad told them incredible stories of his journeys and were intrigued to find out reality wasn't far off. A few showed interest in reading the book.

In December, I debated sending Dad a card. Keith, Jackie, and I agreed to send two more boxes of chocolate and, for the first time, to make sure the nurses told him it was from his three children. Turned out he didn't say much more than thanks to the staff.

Christmas was around the corner. I bought chocolate-covered cherries—one box for each of my siblings and my kids—in honor of Dad. These confections reminded us of childhood holidays, a familiar gift underneath the Christmas tree.

On December 25, 2018, after the boys opened their presents and gorged on candy, the house was quiet. I sat with Leo in my bedroom.

"I'm thinking of calling Dad," I said.

"You should," Leo said. "Why wouldn't you?"

"What if he doesn't want to talk to me? What if he's angry? Or doesn't remember me?"

"How will you know unless you call?"

He was right. What's the worst that could happen? Things would stay the same as they had been for the past ten years. If nothing else, if I could hear his voice, I could confirm he was off the streets. Ultimately, that's what mattered most—his safety.

I brought my sons into my bedroom and told them to standby to possibly speak to their grandpa. Justin hadn't seen him in years, but remembered sharing a bunk bed at the age of five with a grandpa who told him fiery demons under his bed were coming to drag them both to hell.

Good times.

David had never met his grandpa and until this moment hadn't even considered he had a living grandfather. He knew about his grandpa's mental illness and walked in annual NAMIWalks to raise awareness. He knew my book showed how mental illness impacted the entire family. He just hadn't been cognizant that he was part of that family.

I dialed the facility number then hung up. What was I going to say? My boys stood around impatiently.

I phoned again and asked the receptionist if I could speak with a resident. She let me know that it would be a while until a nurse could get him on the phone. She put me on hold.

I clung to the minutes as a comfortable distance.

At last, I heard a faint, shaky voice, but with the familiar Chicago accent. "Hello?"

CHAPTER SIX

Found

"Dad?" I paused, afraid I'd frighten him away. "It's Amanda."

He was quiet. Then, "Hello, Amanda."

Like normal—well, schizophrenia flat-emotion type of normal. As if nothing was out of the ordinary here.

"Do you remember me?" I asked.

"Yes," he said, his voice a little hoarse.

I nodded to my sons and gave them a thumbs up.

Dad had said my name. He had acknowledged my existence. He remembered me. I didn't detect anger or confusion nor did I sense happiness or joy. This is one of the symptoms of schizophrenia—the absence of emotion.

"It's been a long time," I said. "Do you remember when we last talked?"

"No."

"Do you remember Keith and Jackie?"

"Yes."

"Do you remember living in West Virginia with Hilda?"

"No."

After asking several more questions, I sighed. Dad had developed a lot of gaps in his memory ever since he got sick. On the bright side, if he had lost his memory this meant he harbored no ill will towards me on account of my book. I knew better than to ask.

"I miss you," I said. "I wanted to tell you I love you."

"I love you, too." His voice had a slight quiver.

"Do you remember your grandson, Justin?"

"Yes."

"He's twenty-two now."

I waited for a response but got none.

"He wants to say hi to you," I said.

"Okay."

I handed the phone to Justin, who, with his Asperger's, was never much of a conversationalist with those he wasn't close to.

"Hi Grandpa," Justin said. "I miss you… I love you." He looked up at me and shrugged, then handed the phone back.

"Dad, your other grandson, David, wants to say something, too. I gave him the phone.

"Hi, Grandpa… I hope to see you soon… Love you."

I put my ear back to the phone. "Dad, I'm so glad we found you and that you're safe. Is it okay if I call you back another time to talk?"

"Yes, that would be okay." Every word seemed to require effort for him to utter.

"I have to go." I didn't know what else to say. "But I'm so glad we found you. Merry Christmas, Dad. I love you so much."

"I love you, too."

That was it.

Dad had been found.

And it was almost exactly ten years to the day, back on December 23, 2008, that I last heard his voice on the phone. Ten years of not knowing if he were alive, and, against all odds, holding on to hope that he was. Even though I wasn't religious any more, my prayers had been answered.

Still, I didn't cry. I mostly felt nothing at all. This wasn't how I thought it would be. I couldn't figure it out. Shouldn't I be happy? Filled with joy? Or had I cried so much that there was nothing left?

The feeling of relief was so fleeting. Back to business—to build a relationship with the new staff, regain Dad's trust—however fickle that was—and to eventually, possibly, meet him in person. Perhaps. I wasn't even sure if the urge to see him was in me anymore. The father I'd found was a stranger—the same stranger who took over his body when his brain went haywire.

What did I expect? There was no reason to still hope. My dad was gone forever.

But maybe not.

Maybe, deep down in the dark recesses of his brain, there were synapses there that remembered the before times, before age fifty-three, before the mental illness. I decided that's what I was setting out to rekindle—any remnants of Dad. I didn't know if that part still existed, or how I'd recognize it if it did.

It had been a long and difficult journey to find him. Years earlier, on Thursday, October 13, 2011, I finally contacted the police to enlist their help in locating him. Before the end of the day, there was an Orange County Sheriff standing in my living room. He was an older man, sturdy build with gray hair, perfect posture, and squeaky leather boots.

"We got a call," he said. "What's the issue?"

I glanced at the gun in his holster. "I want to make a missing persons report."

He pulled out a pen and paper. "Who's missing?"

"My dad."

"When's the last time you've seen him, and do you know where he may be?"

It had been years and I told him so. I explained his severe mental illness.

The officer didn't write anything down. He glanced up at me. "What do you hope to accomplish?"

"To find him."

"Why?"

"To get him in treatment." What I didn't say aloud was that I knew this outcome wasn't possible if he wasn't alive.

He shook his head. "I see these cases all the time. We pick 'em up. Drop 'em off at the hospital. Then they're back on the streets."

"The revolving door of jails and hospitals," I said. I had been speaking in front of audiences on the very topic for years. "I'm sorry. That must be frustrating."

"Not really," he said with a stone face. "Used to it."

His callousness surprised me.

He cleared his throat. "Even if you file the report, what's going to change?"

"Haven't you heard of Laura's Law?"

He gave a puzzled look.

"Assisted Outpatient Treatment," I said. "Paid for by Prop 63, modeled after Kendra's Law in New York. It's been proven to save money and lives. I wonder why they haven't offered you training on the new law." Bold statement perhaps, but I kept going. "So, yes, I want to report my dad missing."

"Haven't heard of it." He held the pen to his notepad. "What's his name?"

I had hoped for a hint of compassion, but got none.

After I shut the door, he returned to his job while I returned to my miserable reality, not knowing if Dad was even alive, and pondered: Why can't we treat those with severe mental illnesses (SMIs) and their families with dignity and respect? What got us here?

Perhaps deinstitutionalization was a large part of the problem—evidence that even our best intentions can lead to unintended consequences. The enactment of the Lanterman-Petris-Short (LPS) Act in 1967 sought to "end the inappropriate, indefinite, and involuntary commitment of persons with mental health disorders." This came about because too many patients had suffered from abuses in the system, held against their will without good cause, and some exposed to involuntary shock therapy and even lobotomies.

But rather than fix the system, society shut it down. When state hospitals closed, inpatient beds weren't replaced. Instead, patients were released back into the community. Good for some, but not for all.

As a result, the homeless and jail populations soared. It should go without saying that neither prison nor the streets are appropriate placement for individuals suffering from severe mental illnesses. They would be much better served with humane inpatient housing. But just offering treatment doesn't mean people will accept it, especially because anosognosia complicates things.

Approximately 50% of those with schizophrenia and other severe mental illnesses suffer from anosognosia, a term coined by neurologists to describe a lack of awareness or insight into one's illness. Multiple research studies and analysis of brain scans have demonstrated this condition correlates with abnormalities in the frontal lobe of the brain. Therefore, while stubborn denial is a conscious decision, anosognosia is not. Thus, someone with anosognosia is likely to refuse voluntary treatment, because, in their impaired reality, there is no condition to treat. (For more information, I highly recommend the book I'M NOT SICK, I Don't Need Help! by Xavier Amador, Ph.D. He's a leading expert in the field and wrote the Foreword to my first book.)

Without this knowledge, it's understandable if many people, including the sheriff, get frustrated when people with SMIs don't adhere to treatment and repeatedly relapse. It can be exhausting to deal with.

But it's more than that. Maybe it's also because untreated SMIs like schizophrenia can be scary—angry outbursts, hallucinations, and delusions, someone screaming on the street corner.

Illogical behavior is unpredictable. Unpredictability is uncomfortable. We watch—or look the other way—while they suffer, while they may be victimized, until they are in crisis and attempt to kill themselves, or someone else. By then, the damage is already done.

Why do we wait so long to help? No one would dare tell a woman they wouldn't treat her breast cancer until she was Stage Four. They wouldn't treat a cancer patient as a social pariah. Put this way, the discrimination is clear.

Not long after that meeting with the jaded sheriff, after several months of back-and-forth emails and phone calls with the missing persons division, an officer and I scheduled to meet in January 2012.

I pulled up to the local Starbucks and approached a blonde woman sitting at a cafe table on the patio. What was a plainclothes officer supposed to be wearing?

"Are you…?" I asked.

She nodded.

I was glad she wasn't in uniform. That would've drawn more attention than I wanted.

She tried to be inconspicuous. We exchanged pleasantries while she put on medical gloves and pulled out a cotton swab. "Do you mind doing this here?"

It was not like I knew many people around there.

The cheek swab was fast, easy, and felt insignificant.

"After your brother…" She glanced at a paper. "Keith…gives a DNA sample, we'll be able to upload this into the National Database of Missing Persons, which will help us to—"

"Identify his body." I had no trouble saying it. Even though I hoped it wasn't true, I figured Dad could already be a homeless John Doe in some coroner's office in some Podunk town across the country.

On the other hand, if he was alive, maybe my DNA would help to get him treatment.

Either way, the odds weren't exactly in our favor. I'd mourned his death. We all had.

Yet here I found myself on Christmas morning in 2018, eating chocolate-covered cherries and listening to David playing with his new toys in the living room. Dad had been found, even if the old dad was still lost.

That afternoon, I updated the family. Ever since Hilda had returned to Argentina, it was challenging to reach her. Her internet service wasn't great, she had only a cell phone number, which none of us could connect with, unsure of whether or not she could even receive international calls, and limited texting, mostly through Facebook Messenger or WhatsApp, which I didn't have. I had her address, but she said mail was unreliable and didn't know whether she'd be staying with family in Buenos Aires or out at their beach house, which required driving along dirt roads that could be washed out just to get to the town.

Even though I sent Hilda messages through FB Messenger, I couldn't tell if she was getting them all. Most pics didn't go through. I sent her a Merry Christmas image and told her I spoke with Dad. Hopefully, I'd hear back from her soon.

I told Jackie and Keith that I'd heard Dad's voice to confirm it was him, and he was open to communication.

"I'm not calling," Keith said.

"Not even to say hi?" I said.

"Why?" he said.

Good question. Why? Why was I really doing this? To trigger his memories to help him reconnect broken synapses so he could regain some semblance of his former self?? Out of love or some distorted sense of obligation? What did I hope to regain? To build a new relationship with Dad 2.0? For him or for me?

"I'll call," Jackie said, "but not today. I'm not prepared for that. What's the number?"

In January 2019, when I heard back from Jackie, I was both impressed with my sister and annoyed at myself.

"You talked to him for almost an hour?" I asked. I barely eked out five minutes.

"Yes," she said, "but he had a hard time standing in the hall, so he had to go."

"What do you mean?" I assumed hospitals had phones in the bedrooms. I realized I had no idea what this facility looked like or if he had his own room or anything else.

"There's a shared phone in the hallway and he has to stand to use it."

"Maybe we can ask them to give him a chair. Did he know who you were?"

"Yes." She paused. "But he seems to be missing a lot of his memories." She listed off half a dozen things he remembered and a dozen he didn't.

"You got all that in the first call?"

"Anyways, I told him I'd call him again."

"I can't believe he talked to you that long. How come he had nothing to say to me?"

"Well," she said, "it was mostly me doing the talking."

After that, both Jackie and I had had several conversations—mostly one-sided—with Dad. I discussed future plans to fly out to Chicago with both of my sons. We would wait until June, after school was out, which would mark thirteen years since I'd actually seen Dad in person. That was back in July 2006, well before David was born.

Time and distance didn't make much of a difference anymore. Just having gotten the chance to tell Dad "I love you" on the phone was far more than I ever expected would happen. Being able to see him in person would be a gift, especially to do so with my boys.

Even though summer was four months away, I researched hotels and priced airfare. Justin was looking forward to seeing his grandpa again and exploring Chicago; David didn't know what to expect.

I told them about all the museums I'd show them, the ones my dad had shown me—the Chicago Art Institute, the Field Museum, the Museum of Science and Industry. We went on websites and sorted through the special museum exhibits. I shared old memories of my dad with them. We were getting hyped up for the trip.

But on Monday, February 25, 2019, a phone call changed everything.

PART TWO

CONNECTIONS (2019)

CHAPTER SEVEN

HEART ATTACK

February 25, 2019, late on a Monday afternoon, when I got home from work, a call came through from Chicago. I had become accustomed to checking the caller ID and answering Chicago calls, even before I found Dad, in hopes of hearing news from or about him.

"Amanda?" Speaking rapidly with a thick West African accent, concern evident in her voice, the woman identified herself as a nurse from his facility. "Your dad is going to the hospital. Ambulance is on the way."

I had trouble processing what she was saying. "Why? What happened?"

"His vitals… not good… blood pressure…his heart… heart attack maybe."

Heart attack? I had difficulty understanding her.

March 2005 flashed through my mind. That's when I got an unexpected call from Dad. I hadn't heard from him in several months at that point and had to decipher his mumbling on the phone. He said he was going into open-heart surgery and that the surgeon made him call me. Dad had had a massive heart attack, the second in less than five months. Severe blockage. Fifty/fifty chance of surviving the procedure. Should he choose not to go under the knife?—The Doctor told me it was one hundred percent chance of death.

And here we were again. Were we about to repeat the past? I sat down on the edge of my bed.

"Can I talk to him?" I asked. "Is he going to be okay?"

"Call Methodist Hospital. Talk to the doctors. Maybe you come here."

"When? I'm in California."

"Oh, not good. I don't know." She gave me the name and number of the Methodist Hospital. "Maybe good if you come now. Joseph is not well."

With a pen and pad of paper in hand, I phoned the Emergency Room at the hospital, but they said he wasn't there yet. I'd have to wait for answers.

I was more than a five-hour flight away, plus an hour to the airport, an hour to the hospital, plus time at the airport. There was no way. But what if Dad died? That wasn't a possibility I wanted to consider. I had just found him.

I paced my bedroom. Maybe the nurse was overreacting. Maybe it wasn't so serious. But what if it was? Cruel world. Give him back then take him away. Maybe this is why we reconnected—the universe's way of allowing us to say our goodbyes.

I opened my laptop, took a seat at my desk, and tried to call again. At last, I was able to reach a nurse in the Emergency Room.

"The doctor is waiting for some test results," she said. "Cardiac markers in his blood tests are high. Are you on your way?"

"We're in California. Do you think we should go out there?"

"If it was my dad, I would."

Leo offered to prepare dinner for me and the boys, so that I could focus on my dad. I phoned my brother.

"What are you going to do?" Keith asked. "Does Hilda know?"

"Get there somehow," I said. "I sent her a message through Facebook, but I don't know if she got it yet. Should I tell Jackie? She'll be devastated."

"Maybe, but she'll make her own decision on what to do."

Unfortunately, when I got in touch with Jackie, it was a day when her anxiety was already sky high.

Her voice quivered. "Yes, I'll go. But I can't... I can't deal with making plans to buy the tickets. I can't handle that right now. I don't want to fly alone. I'm too upset."

"Don't worry. I'll figure out the plane tickets." I typed away on my computer as we talked. "Okay, I can fly from L.A. on Alaska Air with a stopover in San Francisco to join you. Then we can fly on American nonstop to Chicago together. That will be less stressful for you if we fly there together."

"Oakland airport is better. Every time I fly in or out of San Francisco, my flights are delayed from the fog or something."

"There aren't any seats available through Oakland. Not tomorrow."

She took a deep breath. "I'll call Tony to see if we can stay with him." Tony was one of her two brothers who had the same mom as her but who weren't related to Keith or me. I knew Tony lived in the Chicago area.

"I'll reserve my tickets," I said. "I'll book through Alaska Air, which departs from LAX at 9:30 AM and arrives in SFO at 11 AM. You get the ticket on American Airlines that departs San Francisco at 2:30 PM and arrives at O'Hare at 8:50 PM. We'll take that flight together."

"You're flying on two different airlines?"

"It's the only thing available. I'm booking through the Alaska Air website. Don't worry. We'll leave SFO on American Airlines on the same plane. When I get to the airport, I'll see if they can change our seats so we can sit together."

"I hate getting to SFO, but it's worth it if we can fly together."

I arranged a substitute to cover my classes at school and for my ex-husband to take care of David.

"Babe," I said to Leo, "Can you get my luggage from the garage?" At over six-feet tall, he didn't need to use the stepladder like I would've.

Leo returned with my burgundy Samsonite Softside Carry-on. He rolled it over to the bed and gave me a hug. "Do you need anything else? I'll keep an eye on Justin and make sure he's fed. Well, him and the dogs."

"I forgot about the dogs. Thank you."

"You have enough on your mind." He gave me another squeeze before leaving me alone to pack. I unzipped the bag and piled in clothes while I made more calls.

I reached out to the hospital staff again. They had moved Dad into a room. I was transferred to talk to his nurse in the ICU. "My sister and I fly out tomorrow from California. We'll get there as soon as we can."

"I need your phone number. I'll have the doctor call you."

I hung up and a few minutes later I had Jackie back on the line. "Tony said we can stay with him. He can pick us up from the airport."

"Great, but we need a rental to get out to the hospital as soon as we land. Let's just figure that out when we get there. I need to finish packing." I pulled my bathroom bag out from underneath my sink.

"I called the hospital and talked to Dad," she said, "but he sounds groggy and out of it."

"You got a hold of him?" Geez, she was good. "Okay let's get some rest. I'll call you in the morning when I get to the airport." I checked to make sure my toothbrush and hairbrush were packed.

I had just finished zipping up my luggage and putting it down on the floor when a cardiologist from Methodist Hospital phoned me.

"Tomorrow?" he said. "You can't get here sooner?"

"It's the first flight out we could get."

"We did an EKG and checked his troponin levels. They're at thirteen and rising."

"I don't understand. What's a normal level?"

"Normal is under one."

I grabbed my pad of paper and pen to take down notes. "Then what does thirteen mean?"

"It indicates an Acute Myocardial Infarction."

"A what?"

"A heart attack."

Fuck. Not again. Why didn't he come out and say that in the first place? Like he assumes I understand medical jargon. "What's going to happen?"

"His enzymes are elevated. We did an EKG. We gave him some medication to lower his blood pressure, including aspirin, and a blood thinner. I want to operate—"

"Can you wait for us?"

"Well, how soon can you be here?"

I glanced at my luggage. "We're flying from California and we want to see him first."

He sighed. "It depends how the numbers look in the morning. Call the hospital when you're on your way here, just in case."

He didn't add what he meant by "just in case."

I slumped down on the carpet, traced my fingers along the worn fabric of my bag, and closed my eyes.

CHAPTER EIGHT

Delayed

On Tuesday, February 26, the early morning rush hour traffic from Orange County to Los Angeles was heavy. I barely found a parking spot at a structure near LAX by 7:30 AM. But the shuttle was taking forever. I tapped my foot while I recalculated the time. If the security line wasn't an hour long, I should be at the gate at least an hour early, thirty minutes before boarding. God, I hated cutting it so close.

The hiss of the brakes alerted me to the shuttle's arrival. After I maneuvered my luggage onboard, I saw I missed some text messages from the airlines. One announced a gate change for my first flight. Okay, fine. That saves time to know now. The other announced a delay in the second flight out of SFO. Just as Jackie predicted. I took a deep breath. It would be fine.

While the bus sat at a long red light, I stared out the window. The airport was in sight. My phone vibrated in my pocket with a call coming through from Jackie.

"This... this can't be happening." I could barely understand her. Panic jumbled up her words. "What are we going to do?"

"Slow down," I said. "What's the big deal? It's just a little delay."

"Delay? Our flight was canceled."

"No, it's not. I got a text that it's delayed."

"Check again."

I looked at my messages. "It says it's delayed."

"Well, I hate to tell you, but you're wrong. I told you we should've gone through Oakland."

The bus roared through a noisy intersection and I raised my voice. "Look, I can't hear you well. I'll call you when I get to the airport."

"I'm already on the airport shuttle. Call me. I can't deal with this."

The line at the Alaska check-in counter snaked back or forth in the queues. While I stood there waiting, I phoned the customer service phone number. The wait time was longer than expected, the machine announced. Yeah, actually that was exactly what I expected. I held the phone to my ear and waited to see whoever could help me first. Minutes ticked by. Finally, I reached the front counter, so I hung up the phone.

"My sister says my connecting flight out of SFO to ORD was canceled."

"Reservation number?"

Sure enough, she was right.

"Why didn't they notify me?" I said. "I need to rebook for me and my sister."

"It's on American Airlines."

"Yes, but I booked it through you."

She shook her head. "I can't access their system. You'll have to head over to the American Airlines help desk or call customer service."

"I was on hold. No one answered."

"Sorry, but I can't help you."

I grabbed my bags and hurried down to the American Airlines terminal. The line at the check-in counter was longer than the one at Alaska. I looked down at my watch. My first flight to SFO was boarding in an hour. Jackie kept frantically calling but I couldn't help her yet. I told her to get in the customer service line over there and together we'd figure it out.

Finally, it was my turn to explain the dilemma to another counter agent.

"I'm sorry," he said. "We can't help you. You didn't book the flight through us."

"But the other airlines said they couldn't help me and sent me here."

"Have you tried the customer service number?"

"I was on hold forever. No one answered."

"Maybe try the help desk?"

"I have to get to Chicago. Please."

"Well, I can book you a new flight, but later you'll have to deal with whoever you booked the first flight with." He tapped the keys on his computer. "If you get to SFO today, we may be able to book two tickets from SFO to Chicago for Wednesday."

"I can't wait until Wednesday. My dad needs me there now. He's in the hospital and—"

"I don't have two seats available today."

I squeezed my eyes shut and balled my fists. Don't scream at him. It's not his fault he can't help. Maybe I should just get up to San Francisco and figure it out with Jackie there.

I moved over to the long TSA security line and dialed customer service again. As the line inched up, I listened on the phone for a sign of hope. Nope. Still on hold. I peered around the shoulders of the people in front. *Longer than expected wait times.*

I put my shoes in the bin and slid my bag across the rollers at the TSA checkpoint.

"You need to put the phone in a tray," a TSA officer said.

I carefully set it down and watched it disappear through the flaps on the conveyor belt.

After going through the body scanner—lift your arms overhead like you're escaping from a hostage negotiation—I gathered my coat and scarf. Chicago would be freezing cold in February. I held the phone to my ear. I was still on an obnoxious hold.

I inquired at the Alaska Airlines gate.

"I can't do anything," the agent explained, "but there's an American Airlines customer service desk down that way. They should be able to help you. But San Francisco is a mess right now. Lots of flights are being canceled. Are you going to board this flight?"

"Do you have anything straight to Chicago either from here or from SFO?" I pleaded, but she shook her head. "Okay, just cancel this flight. There's no point in me wasting time getting stuck up there instead of down here."

She tapped away at her computer. "Okay. I canceled this one. Good luck. I hope you find something."

So did I. I headed back to get in yet another line of frustrated travelers. My stomach growled. I hadn't eaten all morning.

The man at the counter clicked away at his computer. "The next few flights are fully booked. But I do have two seats on a red eye from here to Chicago."

"You do? Oh my gosh. Thank you."

I texted my sister:

> Get a flight to LAX. I can get us from here to Chicago tonight.

The agent cleared his throat. "Before they disappear, do you want to book these?"

"Yes." Everything would finally be okay now. Thank the universe.

"Hmm… I'm having a problem getting your sister booked. It says she already has a flight booked?"

"What? No, our flight from SFO was canceled."

"She's not on your reservation. Did you book her original flight?" I shook my head.

"Oh. She needs to get them to release her from whatever flight they have her on. Until then, I can only get a ticket for you. Do you want this one?"

"No, I can't leave without her. Can you give me a second?" I stepped to the side.

Here I was stuck at LAX with no flight to Chicago. What the fuck was happening?

Before I could call Jackie, my phone rang. It was Chicago.

A woman announced himself as the nurse from the hospital who I'd spoken to the previous day. I asked her for an update on Dad's condition.

"Your dad is normally alert and oriented, times three," she said. "Today he's times one. He's weak, can't walk, muffled speech. The doctor wants to get your dad into surgery. Are you on your way to the hospital?"

I didn't want them to operate before Jackie and I could see him first, just in case the surgery wasn't successful. We needed to at least tell him we loved him after all these years of him being gone. That's what I believed the universe wanted for us all, to reconnect, to make peace.

I explained the travel nightmare to the nurse. "Please, can't you wait?"

"We'll monitor him. Call when you arrive. I don't know how long the doctor will wait."

Things were getting too complicated. I messaged my sister:

> Change of plans. I couldn't get your ticket. Don't come here. Get to Chicago. ORD or Midway. Doesn't matter. Just get to Chicago.

I turned back to the gate agent and asked him to book me on the red eye in the meantime. I tapped my foot while I waited. My pocket vibrated. It was Jackie phoning.

"Amanda," she said. I could tell she'd been crying. "I finally got a flight booked to Chicago. It arrives at O'Hare at nine."

"Finally, some good news."

"You don't know what I went through to get that. I had a breakdown at the counter. I was crying and told her it would be on her hands if Dad died before I could get there. She was so snippy. It wasn't until I screamed that my dad was dying and everybody was staring that she even pretended to care."

I pushed back the visual of Dad dying on an operating table. "Did you get through security?"

"Yes, I'm at my gate."

"I could only book a redeye."

"Can't you get there earlier? I don't want to figure out the rental car. Never mind. I'll have Tony pick me up. At least we'll get to the hospital in the morning."

Okay at least we had a plan in place. Things were going to work out. We'd get there. Dad would be fine. I repeated these thoughts until I believed them.

I scoured the terminal for a place that still served hot breakfast. I sat by myself at a table and forced myself to eat. I buttered my English muffin and texted Leo an update on the chaos and drama. At least I'd be there by the morning. I focused on enjoying my scrambled eggs and crispy bacon.

My phone rang, again. Again, it was Chicago.

"Is this Joseph's daughter?" the man asked. "I'm a nurse at Methodist Hospital."

"Yes?"

"Are you almost here? Your dad is not doing well."

"I'm still in California, but I'll be there by the morning."

He was quiet for a moment. "You can't get here sooner?"

"Why?" Half-joking, I added, "He's not going to die, is he?"

He gave a long pause. "We're not miracle workers. We're doing what we can. I can't make any promises."

I dropped my fork. I heard nothing but looked around at the mostly empty dining area. Commuters rushed by with their luggage, businessmen and women, flight attendants, a dad holding a baby, a mom herding a little girl.

Dad might die. It wasn't a joke. It was a real possibility.

Maybe I should call back and tell them to go ahead and operate. But what if he didn't make it? What if this were my only chance to tell him I loved him in person? How horrible for him to have been so utterly alone for ten long years, consumed by mental illness, roaming the streets, confined in a facility, to never hold his children, to never have a single hug from a loved one for ten … long … years. To be so completely alone. To die alone.

This was the dad who always kissed us goodnight and said, "I love you" before we went to sleep, who turned out the lights, who creaked open Jackie's bedroom door to check on us several times. The same dad whose face lit up when he came home from work, still in his suit and tie, and I grabbed ahold of his legs trying to trip him in play, until he'd pick me up, and I'd hug him tight, and he'd squeeze me back. Yes, this was my dad.

He wouldn't die a stranger on the streets, but he'd die alone nonetheless.

I phoned Leo. By the time he answered, tears were streaming down my face.

"Oh my God." I sobbed. "I don't know if I'm seeing Dad or preparing for his funeral."

Leo tried to make me feel better, to tell me there was hope, but there wasn't much he could do. I appreciated his "I love you" and wished I'd have the opportunity to say the same to my dad.

After we hung up, I sat there in silence.

CHAPTER NINE

Now Boarding

I NEEDED TO get to Chicago. Now. The red eye flight would arrive too late. Even though I doubted I could find a seat on an earlier flight, I had to try.

I dumped the rest of my food and got back in the customer service line, which snaked back and forth into the main corridor, filled with frustrated travelers, most of whom were dealing with canceled flights. The line inched up, even with several agents working the counter. I felt the tension and negative energy around me.

If I did get there on time, would Dad recognize me? Would I recognize him?

I remembered how he had appeared as a stranger when I picked him up from the Greyhound Station in Anaheim, California so many years ago. An agency in Atlanta, Georgia gave him a one-way ticket out west, to reduce their homeless population by one. The man who walked through the parking lot had on a blue polo shirt, jeans with a leather belt, and only a small backpack slung on one shoulder. I did not recognize him then … until I looked into his clear blue eyes. That was the window into what remained of my dad, the sliver of hope.

Housing Dad in my place only lasted two months before he was back on the streets. I had provided him with food and clothes and a place to sleep, but after he lashed out at me and my then five-year-old son with unpredictable temper and his manipulative lies, I had to kick him out. I felt awful, but I had to choose my son's safety over my dad's—a horrible choice to have to make. He was an adult. I couldn't legally control him, even if he couldn't control himself.

The line in front of me moved up.

I draped my heavy coat over the handle of my luggage and rolled it forward. I shifted my weight from one leg to the other. My feet were going numb from all the standing.

Was this Dad's third heart attack? Or were there ones I didn't know about? What if Dad refused to see me like he did to Hilda after his open-heart surgery?

At last, it was my turn at the counter.

"I'm sorry ma'am," the agent said. "With so many delayed and canceled flights, you're lucky we can get you there tomorrow."

"Tomorrow isn't good enough." I held back my tears. "My dad's in the hospital."

"Everything is completely sold out."

"It's a medical emergency. You can call the hospital to confirm. My dad's having a heart attack. The doctors keep calling. He may die before I get there. I haven't seen him in ten years. He was homeless and missing and I just found him. Please help me. I need to see him alive."

The man gave me a sympathetic look and tapped at his keyboard. "Maybe we can get you on standby. Maybe someone didn't make a connection. What flight do you want me to check?"

I hadn't even looked up the options. I glanced at the gate on my right. On the screen it said "Now Boarding." The destination: Chicago. Arrival time: 9:23 PM.

"That one." I pointed.

"Hold on, let's see what I can do… you're not going to believe it, but I have one middle seat in the last row. Do you want it? I need to book it quickly before someone else does."

"Yes. A million times, yes." I took a slow breath as tears wet the corners of my eyes. "Thank you so much. I can't thank you enough."

He handed me a printed ticket. "Go get on your flight." He smiled. "Good luck with your dad."

The gate agents called the final boarding group.

I texted my sister an update with instructions not to go to her brother's. I told her we'd rent a car and head to the hospital together. What I wondered, but didn't text, was whether or not Dad would be alive by the time we arrived.

The flight attendants announced there wasn't any room left in the overhead bins, so those of us in line would have to gate-check our bags. I groaned, but did so, appreciative to even be on this flight.

My phone battery was low and there weren't any open plugs, so I tucked it in my pocket and waited for the people ahead of me to board. It rang, again. Chicago.

I whispered into the phone. "This is Amanda."

It was the cardiologist from the hospital. "When will you be here?"

Why was I getting the same question a million times? What part of my answer was not being understood? I thought for a moment. After I land, it would probably take at least half an hour to debark and get my bag, thirty to forty minutes to catch a shuttle to the rental car garage, then time to rent a car, one hour to drive into the city. "Maybe midnight? How are his…" I looked down at my notes on my phone. "His troponin levels?"

"In ER, he was thirteen. In ICU he was twenty-six. Now, he's at thirty and it's rising. Come straight to the hospital. It doesn't matter how late. His surgery will be the first one in the morning." He paused. "Get here as soon as you can."

Hell, if I had wings, I would've been there already.

I texted Jackie. She texted that she was turning off her phone because her flight was getting ready to taxi and she was scheduled to land at 9:15 PM. We couldn't believe our good fortune—we'd be there at the same time.

I sat back in my seat, elbows tucked against my sides, and closed my eyes. I focused on the air blowing on my face.

God, I haven't prayed to you in a long time, and frankly, probably don't still believe in you, but if you are real, please, please, please, keep my dad alive.

CHAPTER TEN

Arrival

I WAS EXHAUSTED but couldn't sleep. I remembered the first flight I had taken. I couldn't have been older than six. My dad, Hilda, Jackie, Keith—he was a toddler—all boarded a flight to Chicago to visit my grandparents and bring Jackie to visit her mom who lived there.

The trip had been a surprise. My sister and I thought we were embarking on another annual road trip. We were quite confused when Dad pulled into a local airport.

"Where are we going?" I asked.

Dad held a finger to his lips and pointed out the window. I had never been on a plane before; I'd only seen them on TV. They were so much bigger up close.

We walked up to the gate—there wasn't much airport security back in 1984—and I pressed my face against the huge glass windows. I still couldn't believe I'd be getting inside a real plane. The roar of the jet engines was nothing like the growl of cars on the streets.

We sat in big padded seats and everyone, not just first class, were served hot meals on large trays. The flight attendant handed us blankets and gave me and my brother a toy plane when I told her it was my first time flying.

The next morning, after dropping Jackie off at her mom's house, Dad drove me, Hilda, and Keith through the outskirts of the city. He pulled off the road and parked in an empty parking lot hidden amongst tall, leafy trees.

"It's a forest preserve," he explained. Then he lifted my three-year-old brother into his arms, and took my hand in his. He led us along a winding path. I looked back for the car, but it had disappeared behind the trees.

"Where are we going?" I asked. Patchy sections of sunlight and dancing shadows of leaves decorated the trail.

"A short hike." It would be the first of many I'd take with him.

"Why?"

"Look around," he said. "Notice all the birds and the trees? If you're really quiet, you can hear them."

The ambient traffic noises had disappeared, replaced by chirping and wind rustling through the leaves. Gravel crunched beneath our feet. Squirrels scurried up thick tree trunks.

Dad squeezed my hand in a comforting embrace.

That was the real him—patient, observant, awed by beauty and small details, which he valued in sharing with his loved ones.

Decades later, the memory was still fresh in my mind. I loved those moments with Dad when he taught me to observe the beauty of nature, which, with our busy lives, was all too easy to ignore. Would I ever make any new memories? Would I even speak to him again?

After the plane touched down at O'Hare Airport, I stretched my legs glad to be out of the cramped space—air travel had changed so much in the last thirty years. I ran into Jackie before I could even call her. We had arrived at the same time in the same terminal at adjacent gates.

Without time for more than a hug, we navigated through the massive airport to get to the car rental shuttle pickup. We stood on the people mover belt, both too exhausted to say much other than to discuss the logistics. Bright rainbow colors shifted into patterns along the walls of the corridor and had a calming effect on my mind.

Her brother Tony knew we had landed but that we were going to head to the hospital. He said his place was ready for us when we got there.

We stepped out into the night air to get onto the shuttle bus. The lake blown air whipped my hair into my face, numbed my ears and the tip of my nose. My teeth chattered and even with a heavy coat, scarf, hat, and gloves, it felt like my bones and eyeballs were freezing.

When we got there at 10 PM, the rental car building on Zemke Boulevard was warm and brightly lit with tall ceilings. There weren't any lines at many of the company counters. We walked up to the first and approached the college-aged agent who had her hair pulled back into a tight bun.

"We need a car for a couple days." I smiled back at my sister, because we had finally made it across the country and would be with Dad soon. "We have to fly back on Friday, but we're planning to bring back the car Thursday night."

"We're staying with my brother," Jackie said. "He can bring us back to return the car the night before our flight—"

"We have an early flight on Friday morning," I said. "We don't want to mess around returning the car in the morning, if you're even open that early—"

"I'm sorry," the agent said. "We don't have any economy or standard cars available."

"That's okay," I said. "We'll take what you got."

Jackie leaned over my shoulder. "How much?"

"It's going to be about five hundred dollars," the agent said.

"What?" My sister and I gasped in unison.

"Are you fucking kidding me?" Jackie said. "For two days?"

"You didn't reserve ahead of time, so you don't get that discount," she said. "We don't have many cars left. This is the current daily rate for the vehicles we have on the lot, plus 11.11% concession fee, the 12% state tax, $8 per day CFC, and a couple dollars per day for vehicle license fee, and a few other things. But everything will be broken down for you on the rental agreement. This amount does include the extra hours, which are almost as much as another day. It does not, however, include the refueling fee, insurance, or tolls, which will be extra."

"That's ridiculous," Jackie said. "What is it? A Maserati?"

"Come on," I said. "Let's try a different company." I turned back to the agent. "Thank you for your help. We'll be back if we change our minds."

"Okay. We close at midnight."

Each counter we went to had a similar price. Same story: sold out, taxes and fees, high demand, we didn't order ahead of time, higher price to rent on the spot.

"Unreal," I said. "It's never cost this much before." I didn't have the money saved up for this unexpected trip. Money was tight at home. I loved my dad, but man, this price tag was killing me.

It was after 10:30 PM by the time we got into line at the last counter. After the customer in front of us signed agreements and walked away, the twenty-something brunette in a turtleneck motioned to us. "Hi. May I help you?"

Jackie rested her elbows on the counter which now supported her head. With hair disheveled, mascara smeared, and tears in her eyes, she explained our plight and summarized what it took for us to get there. "I don't want my dad to die." She took a shaky breath. Her voice quivered. "Please, please, is there any discount, AAA, or anything you can possibly do to help us? We need to get to the hospital."

The woman locked eyes with my sister and gave her a sympathetic smile. "I lost my dad not too long ago." She handed Jackie a tissue. "Let me see what I can do." She pursed her lips together and clicked at her keyboard. Then she leaned in closer to us and lowered her voice. "I can get you a car for one hundred and fifteen dollars and twenty-seven cents."

"What?" I said. "How?" At that moment, she might as well have said free.

She patted her hand down to hush us. "I'm going to give you an employee rate and a company discount."

"Oh my God," Jackie started crying. "You're an angel. An absolute angel."

"I feel so bad for you both. Plus, it's starting to snow. Do you need a map or directions on how to get to the hospital?"

I heaved my sister's bag into the back of the compact SUV—what did she bring? rocks? With her anxiety and fatigue, and the snow, we decided best that I drive. I didn't mind. It was so cold I could see my breath. I rubbed my hands together for warmth and, while the car windows defrosted, I phoned the hospital. It was now close to 11 PM.

"We're so glad you made it to Chicago. Don't worry how late it is, hon, come on up. Go in through the ER. We're expecting you."

With heat blasting, we headed east on I-90. I had to drive slowly because of the slippery roads. It was midnight by the time I pulled in the hospital lot, snowflakes were coming fast, the ground dusted in white. Jackie held onto to my arm for support while we navigated patches of ice. The front door sign said visiting hours were over. I motioned to the security guard inside the ER entrance.

He nodded. "You here to see Joseph? You his daughters from California, right?" He buzzed open the next door. "Head on up the elevator."

"I don't know if I can do this," Jackie whispered. "I'm having a hard time right now."

"We're here," I said. "We made it. It's fine." I led her in.

"I haven't seen Dad in a long time. I don't know if I can handle it."

I didn't know what to say to her. It had been just as long for me, yet I wasn't allowing myself to fall apart over it. I squeezed her hand.

When the elevator doors opened, two female nurses, one half the age of the other, greeted us with warm smiles. The area was well lit but silent, other than occasional beeps and hums.

"We're so glad you made it here," the older one, a brunette with short curls and a kind smile, said. "We were worried you wouldn't get here in time."

"What time does he go into surgery?" I asked.

"An ambulance will pick him up around six-thirty."

"Why? Where's he going?"

"We need to transfer him to Weiss Hospital for the heart surgery. It's not far from here."

"We'll make sure to make it back here by then," I said.

The two nurses exchanged a glance. "Where are you staying?"

"With my brother in Schaumburg," Jackie said.

"Schaumburg?" the younger nurse, with long black hair and smooth skin, said. "You're not going to make it there and back by the morning. Not with traffic. You won't sleep at all."

The other nurse nodded. "We thought you were staying out here. Tell you what, we're not very busy tonight. We have another bed in his room and we can easily bring in a third. That way you can stay here in the room with your dad."

What angels. I wanted to cry from their generosity and kindness.

"I don't know if that's a good idea," Jackie said. "We haven't seen our father in over ten years. I don't know if I—" She started sobbing. "I—I can't... I can't do this." I wrapped an arm around her, but was too exhausted to offer any more emotional support.

"Honey, have a seat. Your dad is sleeping right now anyways. Have you eaten anything?"

"Not since breakfast," I said.

One of them ushered us down a hallway and into a room. A table, a couple chairs, a counter, and refrigerator adorned their break room. "The cafeteria is closed, but we have juice. Do you prefer apple, or cranberry, or both? We can find you something to eat, probably some sandwiches. Help yourselves to anything here."

With all the stress of getting across the country now subsiding and especially with the offer to stay, I felt pressure lift from my shoulders. It was okay to slow down and enjoy a meal.

"I'm craving deep dish pizza," I said, now acutely aware of my hunger. "Does anyone deliver here?"

"It's late, but a few still deliver," the younger one said. "Hold on and I'll get you some menus."

Jackie paced. "I shouldn't have come. This was a bad idea. I can't do this."

I didn't know how to reply, so I was glad when the younger nurse reappeared with the menus.

"Our treat," I said. "We appreciate your kindness."

The delivery took over forty-five minutes—deep dish pizza takes a long time to bake—but Jackie and I were glad to have some time to relax and catch up while we waited. The nurses kept offering us more juice and checking in on us.

"By the way," I told them, "Dad has a severe mental illness and we don't know if he's been taking his medicine."

"Oh, that makes sense." The younger one exchanged a glance with the other.

"I figured as much," the older one said, "when he tore off all of the cables and monitors and wandered into the hallway hollering."

Jackie shook her head and looked away.

"Sorry," I said. "He's not really in his right mind."

"Oh, don't worry, hon. We gave him some apple juice, and got him back into the room."

I was famished by the time the pizza arrived. The nurses went back to doing their rounds.

After savoring a thick slice, I was stuffed, tired, and ready to see Dad. We gave the nurses the rest of the pizza to share with the security guard, which they said he'd appreciate and we headed towards Dad's room. It was now past one in the morning. There was no other reason for delay as far as I was concerned. My sister could do what she wanted.

I followed the nurse into a dark room; Jackie lingered a step behind me. I held my breath for what I'd find as we entered the doorway.

CHAPTER ELEVEN

Recognition

There Dad was, on a bed, in a hospital gown, under blankets, half asleep, connected with tubes and wires, a constant beeping the only sound.

"Joseph," the nurse approached him. "Your daughters are here to see you."

He grunted.

"Do you want to see your daughters? Amanda and Jackie are here."

He nodded. The nurse motioned us over.

"Dad?" I leaned in close, held the tubes out of the way to give him a hug. He didn't move but allowed my touch. "Dad, I love you." I wrapped my arms around him, rested my head on his shoulder, and breathed in the moment. I felt his skin against my cheek. This was my Daddy. I listened to his heart beat on the monitor and pulled away.

His eyes, with their faraway gaze, focused on my face. There was no hint of a smile in his cheeks or at the corners of his eyes, but only the blank expression that schizophrenia had cursed him with. Still, he intently stared at my face. Maybe deep inside, Dad was still there. Maybe all he needed was to be reminded.

"I missed you, Dad." I wiped my eyes. "I'm so glad we found you. We're here now. I'm going to stay with you."

Again, the blank expression, or lack of one. But I detected a tiny nod and he closed his eyes. No hellos, no it's nice to see you, none of the I-haven't-seen-you-in-forever type of greetings. But he had looked me in the eyes. That was recognition.

Was I relieved? Frustrated? Angry? Happy? Intellectually, I was all of those things, but the emotions eluded me. I wasn't sure what I felt, other than numb. Maybe I was too tired to connect with my feelings, or maybe they fled years ago.

I turned. My sister had her hand over her mouth. I couldn't see her well in the darkness, but by her sniffles, I knew there were tears in her eyes. I stepped back and she led me out to the hallway.

"Oh my God, Amanda, did you see him? It's so sad. He looks horrible. Look at all those machines. I can't…"

"Are you going in to see him?"

She shook her head and walked away sobbing. I should have felt sorry for her, but I didn't.

There were so many things I wanted to say to her but didn't: Get it together. We're here for Dad. It's not about us. This wasn't a big surprise. What was she expecting? Did she think Dad was going to jump up, give us a bear hug, and ask us about our trip, laughing and joking about all the mishaps? Was she expecting him to ask about his four grandchildren, Jackie's daughters and my sons, two of whom he'd never met, none of whom knew him? To demonstrate care and concern for our wellbeing, to plan a future vacation with us? God. We'd sooner be struck by lightning than receive any of that. I knew it. She had to have known it.

This is how it was before he disappeared. The dad we knew and loved died slowly beginning in 1996. By 1999, Dad was dead. This was schizophrenia's reproduction of our dad, a clone of his body, but not his mind or heart. Why did she think it'd be any different now?

Perhaps she shouldn't have come.

CHAPTER TWELVE
THE PROPHET

I WAS GLAD when one of the nurses led Jackie away to another room at the opposite end of the hallway. Good. Go cry it out. I stood there in the doorway.

I knew I sounded like a jerk, but I didn't care. Who had tracked Dad down for ten fucking years? Me. Who hadn't given up hope despite everything? Me. Who wrote a Goddamn book about our family's story? Me. What had she done? Gone on with her life. That's it. Yes, consumed with anxiety and depression. But I had depression, too. And I wasn't sitting here feeling sorry for myself. I was the one living in reality.

What I didn't understand, couldn't possibly understand, was how heavy the weight of emotions pressed down on her, how intimately attuned Jackie was to everyone around her, the intensity of the world too much to bear. She couldn't have done what I had. While I thought and planned, she felt and grieved.

But none of that was in the realm of my understanding at that moment. All I felt was irritation and anger. Perhaps some of it was misplaced, but I couldn't care less—instead, my focus was completely on my dad. I went back into his room and returned to his side.

The nurses wheeled in a second medical bed for me, then left to go tend to my sister. Dad turned to look at me, the same vacant look in his clear blue eyes, and studied my face.

I gave him a hug and sat on the edge of his bed. "I never gave up hope in finding you. I've missed you so much." I wiped away the tears and held back the rest. "I missed you. I wish you weren't so sick and that you were back to how you used to be when I was little."

"Amanda." His voice was croaky. "I know things. God has spoken to me."

Why couldn't he be normal? Although incredulous to be near him and relieved to hear his voice again, I couldn't deal with his insanity at the moment. The weight of fatigue weighed heavy on me. I shook my head and retreated to my bed. "God doesn't talk to you." I said this despite knowing better than to argue with someone who had anosognosia, the inability to understand they are ill or their illness. Maybe I shouldn't have said it. "It doesn't matter. You're here now. And I'm here with you. How are you feeling?"

"Not good."

"I'm sorry you're in pain. I'm here now, but I'm exhausted." I slipped underneath the blankets and lay my head on the flat pillow. Sleep would come quickly.

"You know, I'm a prophet."

"You've told me before." I couldn't pry my eyes open any longer.

"I've met other prophets before."

"Really," I said flatly, to humor him. "Where?"

"All living on the streets. Chicago; Savannah, Georgia, different places…They see things, too. God showed them evil people."

"And how did you know they were prophets?"

"I just know…Holy Ghost, you know that you know. You will see things, and hear things, and God shows you."

"Right." I rolled away from him. "We can talk tomorrow. I'm tired."

"I was chased by wild dogs and helicopters sent by the devil. You wouldn't believe it."

That was the truth. "Dad, come on, I need sleep."

"I know things. I've had visions. I've seen heaven, colors are heavenly, beautiful, brilliant colors—"

"Dad, seriously I'm exhausted. If you can't let me sleep, I'll go to the other room." It was surreal. Dad was repeating himself, telling me the stories he'd relayed to me over a decade earlier. Although not the typical stories you'd hear your aged dad or grandpa repeat, it was nonetheless old news to me. My patience was gone. Still, I was strangely comforted to hear his voice, despite the disturbing words flowing through his mouth.

He was quiet for a few minutes. Then he started up again.

"In Ft Lauderdale—I'd seen it in my dreams before—I went into a Haitian church and—"

"And the angels were there singing and dancing in circles before running out of the church and disappearing." I grunted. "I know. You've told me before."

"Singing God's praises. Nobody else saw them. I've had other visions that—"

"Dad, I'm serious. Please stop. I. Need. Sleep." I sighed and rolled back over to face him. I opened my eyes and studied his face. Maybe he was scared of the surgery. Maybe the free flow of his thoughts indicated his fears. No time had passed between us. It was like yesterday that I'd parted from him in Chicago never to hear from him again. But here we were. Side-by-side. In the same room.

He stopped talking and stared up at the ceiling.

"Dad, I love you. I'm so glad to be here with you. We can talk tomorrow. I promise."

With that, I drifted off to sleep.

I awoke to the bustle of nurses in the room. I looked at my phone. It was already well after seven in the morning on February 27, 2019.

"Amanda?" one said. "We're getting ready to transport him. The paramedics are here."

I stretched and sat up, wearing the same clothes as yesterday. I remembered where I was and how I got there. "Where's my sister?"

"She's waiting in the hallway. Will you be riding in the ambulance?"

"Let me talk to Jackie." I reunited with her. Her eyes were red and puffy.

"I didn't sleep much," she said," but there's no way I could've slept at all in there with him."

"Only one can ride in the ambulance with him," a paramedic said. "Who's coming?"

Jackie shook her head.

"I can," I said, "if you can drive the car there."

"Not in the snow, I can't. I haven't had enough sleep."

And I had? I would've preferred to have one of us with him, but chose not to push the issue. "Okay, we'll follow in our car." I patted Dad's arm. "We'll meet you there."

They wheeled Dad out. He was quiet, his face without emotion. He closed his eyes.

CHAPTER THIRTEEN

VITALS

It was 8:45 AM. Nurses were busy trying to start a second IV in Dad's right hand by the time my sister and I made our way to his bedside at Weiss Memorial Hospital.

Dad chatted while everyone worked and filled out paperwork.

Jackie recorded Dad on her phone while I stood by and observed the two of them conversing. Neither of us knew if this would be the last time that we'd see Dad alive. Not to mention, if it were on video, it might make it more real to us.

"When I was an infant in my crib," Dad said, "I saw a scary face looking at me. And later on, I found that was the devil. He had occurred many times in my life. I believe in the devil. I believe in heaven. I believe in both. Jesus come to me in a dream ten times. Looks exactly—"

"But when did you first see Jesus?" Jackie interrupted. "When you were an infant?"

"I had dreams when I was young. But especially after I…yeah, and I didn't know the Bible. I had a dream and everything was a bright light and there was a glowing disc behind it. Then when I started to read the Bible, decades later, it said there was no need for the sun and the moon for the glory of God did enlighten it and the lamb was the lamp thereof. So, it came to me, I didn't come to it. It wasn't because I read the Bible... I had no religious training."

"And what color did you say heaven looked like to you?" Jackie asked.

"It was many different colors."

"So, do you feel at peace right now? Do you want to go to heaven?"

"I'll go to hell."

"No, you won't. No, you won't."

"Yeah, because when I was in the early days at the facility, I was sitting at a table on the first floor and a woman sat down at the table. I never saw her before, and I knew everyone in the building, not by name. And I told her a lie, which wasn't the first time lied. And she said, 'you're going to hell' and she walked away. And starting when I went back to my room, at dark, a shadow came across everything. And all my dreams and visions stopped."

"But you know what... that woman was a patient. She was ill. Her curse was not real, Dad. You're going to heaven because you're a good person."

"No, I'm not a good person."

"Yes, you are. You have never killed anybody. You have never hurt anybody, physically."

"But I talk too much."

"Oh, who doesn't." Jackie smirked. "Amanda and I talk a lot, too. I used to get in trouble at school."

"I wasn't, I wasn't on drugs. I wasn't hallucinating. I wasn't lying. I wasn't misinterpreting. And these things I saw really did happen. It isn't me. But other people have seen them, too."

"Oh. You know what? I knew that something was happening to you on Sunday. I got a phone call on Monday from Amanda and I felt something on Monday morning when I woke up, and I said, I've got to talk to Dad. And a couple hours later, the phone rang and Amanda said, 'Jackie, you need to get on a flight from California as soon as possible to Chicago.' So, I think God was telling me I needed to be here. I knew something was happening the day before it happened. So, I believe. I do believe there's something out there talking to us. And you're safe."

"Yeah, you're only going to know at the end. 'Cause we're not going to get out of this world. It's getting into the next one. And many people believe different things, some people don't believe, and other people believe as much as they don't believe."

"But you know you're safe, okay. And you're going to the pretty heavens."

"Yeah, I wasn't always…and there were a lot of things they did to me, which wiped out my memory. And I was in strange situations."

"Who wiped out your memory?"

"I don't know. But they could do that with drugs or hypnosis or whatever. I don't know the technology."

"Do you remember—"

"But my memories are very technical but I do know—"

"Do you remember that I'm your daughter?"

"Huh?"

"Do you remember that I am your oldest daughter? I'm Jackie. Do you remember me? Jackie?"

"Yeah."

"Do you know how old I am now?"

"Probably forty-something."

"You want to look at me?"

"Yeah."

"I'll be forty-seven in April."

"Okay."

"I'm forty-six and Amanda is, oh God, how old is Amanda?"

"Forty-two."

"No, wait…wait, wait… forty-one. Here's Amanda." She spun the camera to me.

"I parked on the street right there," I said to a nurse. "That's safe? That's free? Okay." Then I saw my sister looking at me. I made conversation with Dad about my parallel parking because he's the one who taught me how. "I went back and forth… I was nervous because old cars had bumpers, the rubber bumpers were—"

"My dad," Jackie noted, "when he was in college, used to drive a taxi cab."

"You drove a taxi?" I said.

"Yeah, a little bit," he said.

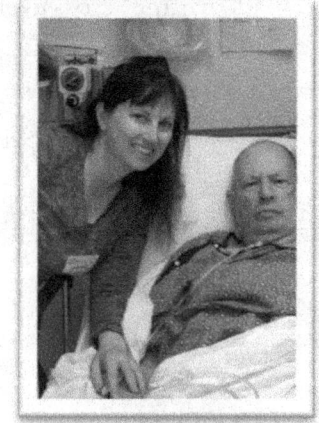

We chatted with the nurses about cab driving before Dad interrupted us. "My whole function now is to give a witness for heaven and hell and all the miracles I've seen that people haven't seen."

Jackie stopped him. "Dad, here's your nurse—"

"Just because you drop a pen on the floor and I say I didn't see that, it's still so. Because you know you dropped a pen. And so, a lot of people don't believe what I say. But I know it's so."

"Dad, this is your nurse, Priscilla."

"I'm only… about spiritual things now."

"Dad, she needs your arm. She's going to take care of you… blood pressure."

"Vitals, you know," Priscilla said.

"Priscilla, where are you from?" Jackie asked. "You have a beautiful accent."

"Ghana."

"I've been to Ghana," Dad said. "I've been to forty countries."

"Is it hot in Ghana?" Jackie asked.

"It's hot," Dad and Priscilla said at the same time.

While Jackie and the nurses talked of families and weather, I complained about my gray hair to Dad, who said gray hair didn't matter to him. A male nurse with a clipboard entered our curtained area.

I took out my phone. "Do you want to see a picture of Justin?"

"I know how Justin looks," he said.

I showed him pictures of my poodle and reminded him of his old poodles, which he said he did remember.

"In my seventy-five years, I've seen so many things. People had miraculous things about heaven and hell that I really believe in that. Because I've had dreams and things that weren't possible for men to stage."

They started on the oxygen and IV's.

"My dad's super smart," Jackie said. "He has a Master's Degree in, what, chemistry?"

"Math," Dad said.

"But he was a chemistry major at Northwestern."

"Yeah, but I'm not that smart."

"You are very smart."

"No, if somebody says something, I know how to parrot it back to them, but I don't have wisdom and it's applying knowledge saying the right thing at the right time to the right person…wisdom… I'm a fool."

"Did you get your Bachelor's Degree in chemistry—"

"A fool—"

"And your Master's Degree in math? I get confused."

"Yeah, I'm not really concerned with this world… just looking forward to the next one."

Jackie and Priscilla discussed school while she adjusted the second IV in Dad's right hand. The male nurse with the clipboard asked a lot of medical history questions. I couldn't answer them even if I wanted to, so I was glad Dad was coherent enough to do so.

"What's the IV for?" Dad asked.

"Well, you're going to have a procedure. And in any procedure, we need a good IV. That other one," he pointed to Dad's left hand," is not working and we need to take it out. Can you stand?"

"I don't know. I'd have to try."

"When's the last time you stood before they took you here?" I asked.

"Yesterday, I stood up. They didn't want me to, but I took everything out and I walked into the hall because I said, 'Where's my meal? I've been waiting for it.' And they made me go back and sit in bed."

"Do you know what the procedure is that you're having done today?" the male nurse asked. "I need you to say it in your own words."

"I don't know. I had a heart attack."

"Dad, the dye test," I said. "To check for blockages."

"What previous surgeries have you had?" the male nurse asked.

"Appendectomy, prostate cancer, open heart surgery—single, not quadruple."

"Any allergies to medications?"

"Sulfa."

"Me, too," Jackie said.

I thought back to a horrible reaction I had in the hospital after one of my two neck surgeries. It was late at night and I was alone in the room. Suddenly, my muscles contracted and it became hard to breathe. I called the nurse and tried not to panic as I felt my arms and legs tighten and breathing became harder. I called again for the nurse and said I couldn't breathe.

A nurse rushed in, disconnected me from tubes and placed me in a seat. She had me swallow a pill and did what reminded me of Lamaze breathing in my face to help me calm. I never knew what caused that frightening reaction, but now I wondered if I too, could have the same allergy as my dad and sister.

As soon as Dad had finished answering the nurse's questions, the male nurse left and a woman with blonde hair and another clipboard entered. At that point, Dad seemed to have a new burst of energy and out of nowhere started telling racist jokes. Jackie and I exchanged horrified glances as Priscilla and the other woman became noticeably uncomfortable.

Priscilla was busy checking Dad's vitals and adjusting tubes and cables, so I pulled the other woman aside. "Can I talk to you for a minute?"

"Sure."

I lowered my voice. "Away from where he can hear."

She led me down the hallway to an empty room.

"Please don't take offense to what he's saying. He's not racist. He's mentally ill. Can you tell the other nurses?"

"Ah," she said. "That makes sense from the things he said when he first got here, before you were here."

I gave her a two-minute summary of my dad's insanity spiral that led a healthy father of three to become an unstable person who roamed the streets and disappeared.

"So, that's where we are," I said. "It's been ten years. Last night was the first time we've seen him since all of that."

She nodded. "Oh, honey. I can't believe you've been through all that. And here you are. You flew across the country on a moment's notice to be by his side. Not many people would do that."

"He was a great dad." Tears I didn't realize I had, came quickly. "I love him."

"It's incredible that after all this time, you never gave up. You still searched for him."

I quietly sobbed; my shoulders shook as the tears slid down my cheeks. "Nobody else on this earth was looking for him, so I figured it had to be me."

CHAPTER FOURTEEN

The Surrogate

I FOUND MYSELF wrapped in this stranger's arms, comforted by her touch.

Crying was cathartic. The feelings I held back for so long—all business, to-do lists, planning, scheduling, writing, calling, writing—were there hiding underneath. And now, they came, all at once.

"It's okay to cry," she said. "You deserve that. You've been through a lot. I'm sure it means a lot to your dad that you're here. Let me know if there's anything I can do for you."

I wiped my arms across my face. She reached over to hand me a tissue and gave me a final hug.

"Thank you," I said. "I didn't realize how much it all affected me."

"I can't imagine it not."

I took a moment to dry my eyes and calm down, to push the emotions back where they came from, at least for now. After a long, deep breath, I headed back to hug Dad goodbye. I got there just as the nurses were unlocking the wheels and pulling open the curtains.

"I love you, Dad," I said and kissed his cheek.

Then I stood alongside Jackie and watched while the nurses wheel him off to his procedure.

My sister and I alternated between pacing the waiting room and sitting side-by-side. She kept glancing at me then pursing her lips.

"You know who should be here?" She plopped down on a seat. "Hilda."

"Why?" I swiveled in my chair to face her. "She's in Argentina."

"Does she even care? Why didn't she move back to California?"

"She's with her sister. Her nieces and nephews and the rest of her family are out there."

"And what about us? We're her family."

"You're busy with your daughters. I'm busy with my boys. Keith is busy with work. What's out there for her besides memories of Dad and all that trauma? She did more for him than anyone and stayed by his side when no one else would have. She was alone."

"But she didn't have to be." Jackie raised her voice. "Hilda made that choice. I could've been there for Dad, but she said everything was fine. That wasn't true. She wasn't being honest."

"Maybe she was trying to protect us."

"That should've been my choice." Jackie crossed her arms and pouted. "Did she even offer to come out here to see Dad?"

"Dad would've refused. Can you imagine how horrible and painful that would've been? He did that to her last time. He refused to even say hi to her after his open-heart surgery. He told her she was from the devil. And what did she do? Spent the whole day with me buying furniture and setting up his apartment so he'd be okay after he left the hospital. Dad didn't thank her. And how about all the other times? When she searched the streets of Chicago for him, alone in the snow?"

Jackie looked away and bowed her head. "She didn't ask for—"

We were interrupted by a loud throat clearing. We both looked up to see a doctor standing over us.

"Are you Joseph's daughters?" he said. "Your dad is doing well. We put in a stent."

"Another one?" I asked. "How bad was it?"

He explained the procedure in detail, answering each of my sister's questions; I didn't care about the nitty gritty. I just wanted him to tell me it was over and was successful.

Dad had a blockage; another stent would buy him some more time. At least they didn't have to slice his chest open and stitch him back together like Frankenstein, as had happened with the open-heart surgery. Perhaps he could avoid another one if he stayed on his medication.

After they sent Dad up to the recovery room—fortunately, he had the room to himself—Jackie fed him his lunch. We draped a towel over his chest, but she kept spilling the juice and getting bread crumbs everywhere. I smirked when she put too much applesauce on the spoon and had to scoop it up after the extra slid down his chin. Dad didn't seem to care, and I thought it funny to watch—like a mother feeding a child for the first time. So, I sat back and let her handle it and checked my messages.

Hilda had responded to me through Facebook Messenger the day before.

> Hello Amanda and Jackie, sorry to hear about your dad, I hope everything will be ok, finally Amandy, you find it, where your daddy is, so many times you told you didn't know, please could let me know how is he doing? call me or I will call you, I'm glad Jackie is with you, how is Keith? God Bless You. I Love you, give him a kiss, his in my prayers

I responded to her:

> Hi Hilda. Jackie and I are in the hospital in Chicago. They just finished Dad's procedure and put another stent in his heart. He did fine and is stable and is recovering in the room right now. He will probably go back to the nursing care home tomorrow.

She replied back:

> How are you, how your daddy doing, is he still in the hospital? I don't think so he's ready to go back to the nursing home, what is plans now, how long are you going to stay there? Let know please, love you

While Dad ate, Jackie and I gave him a Cliff Notes version of the last ten years of our lives. He didn't say much more than grunts and barely noticeable head nods, so we kept chatting, hoping some information would sink in and stick.

After they confirmed Dad would be sent back to the nursing home the following day, Jackie and I decided to visit the rehabilitation facility immediately, to meet the people we'd spoken to so many times on the phone over the past six months.

We had a goal—get Power of Attorney documents filled out. We'd learned a lot about HIPAA and other legal roadblocks and were intent on not repeating the mistakes from the past. Sure, Dad was cooperative now, talking to us both, but tomorrow could be a different day. His unpredictability had been the only predictable part of his mental illness. Before we got there, Jackie had me stop so we could pick up cookies and cupcakes for the staff at both the hospital and the facility.

"Why?" I asked.

"Kindness goes a long way," she said. "Trust me on this."

As we drove through neighborhoods to get to the rehab facility, the area seemed unremarkable, just another part of the brick houses and narrow tree-lined street. But our first impression upon walking up to the place was confusion. Raucous chatter came from the enclosed front patio filled with patients. We crossed the street, greeted by a stank of cheap cigarettes.

Inside, we identified ourselves to the receptionist.

"Oh, honey," the older woman said. "It's nice to finally put a face to the voice."

The director and office employees were nice, especially after Jackie gave them cookies. I asked Jackie to let me meet privately with the person who handled the financial records. Jackie stayed out of the office and chatted with the receptionist while I took a seat at the young woman's desk. She couldn't have been older than twenty-five and eyed me suspiciously.

"How's Dad's stay being paid for?" I asked.

"He's on Medicaid and Social Security." Sounding a bit defensive, she added, "Those funds need to come directly to us."

"Is his pension coming here?"

"His what? I don't know anything about that." She narrowed her eyes. "I'll need that information."

"I don't know the details yet. We just found him." Oh no. Had I said something I shouldn't have? I didn't want to endanger his status. "We're trying to figure everything out. How long is he going to be here for?"

"He's a resident."

"Can I get a copy of his medical records?"

"I can't share that information with you."

"I'm sure he'll give you permission. How long has he been here?"

"I only handle the money."

"You must have at least his admission date in your records."

She stood up and ushered me out the door. "Let's have you talk to the social worker."

She led Jackie and I downstairs to the social services office where, again, the three women inside welcomed us but with an undertone of hesitation. The financial officer waved bye and left the room.

"Can we get the Power of Attorney forms filled out?" I asked. "I'm sure we can get Dad to sign."

"You need a witness," the social workers said. She was an older woman with a tight bun and life-hardened face. "And it needs to be notarized."

"Can you do that?"

"No," she said flatly.

"What about a nurse?"

"No."

"Well then how are we going to get it signed?"

She shrugged. "You might want to consult a lawyer."

"Are you kidding me?" I eyed the two assistants, younger women sitting on unmatched chairs around old metal desks. They didn't respond. I sharpened my tone. "We just flew out here from California to help him. What are we supposed to do?"

"Look," Jackie took over, with a calmer voice. "What my sister and I are needing is some way to make sure you check in with us regarding medical decisions related to our father."

"For that," the social worker explained, "we have a Certification for Surrogate Decision-Making form."

Finally, we were getting somewhere. "Can we see the form?" I asked.

A younger assistant creaked open an old filing cabinet drawer and pulled out some manila folders. "We probably have a paper copy in here somewhere."

Jackie changed the subject. "Do you all know my sister is an award-winning author? She wrote a book about Dad."

"Wow. Really?" the other assistant asked. "What's it called?"

"Do you have a copy?" the social worker asked. "I'd love to hear more."

All three women instantly changed demeanor and broke out in chatter, which Jackie kept going. They all gushed about being avid readers while Jackie hyped up my book.

One of the assistants produced a paper from a folder. "Here it is."

The older woman smiled and pointed at the document. "Which one of you would like to be listed as the surrogate? We can only put down one person."

I looked at my sister. Surely, she would agree that I'd be the best choice. After all, I'm the reason we reunited with him.

"I'm the oldest," Jackie said. "So, it should probably be me."

Rather than argue with her, yet, I said, "Why don't we call Keith and get his opinion? It should be a shared decision."

We got Keith on the phone and Jackie got him caught up on Dad's progress, while the social worker began to fill out the form. For "Decisional capacity," she marked "The resident lacks the capacity to make decisions concerning health care, including life sustaining treatment. The cause and nature of the resident's impairment is related to" and the third box was checked: "Severe, persistent mental illness."

Below that, the next section read, "The resident has a qualifying condition and/or meets the criteria for one or more of the following categories." There were four options. The woman skipped the first three "Terminal Condition, Permanent Unconsciousness, and Incurable or Irreversible Condition."

I mused that his severe mental illness was both terminal and incurable, as well as, unfortunately, irreversible. If only we could go back in time, twenty years earlier. If only there were a cure. If only we could go back to the way that it should have been, with Dad being capable of being a dad and being able to enjoy his later years as a grandfather. But, nope. Fate had denied us all of that outcome.

So, she checked the last box: "The resident does not have a condition listed above <u>but lacks decisional capacity</u> and needs an advocate and representative to make decisions on his/her behalf. *Note - A health care surrogate cannot tell the doctor to withdraw or withhold life-sustaining treatment or consent to an order for such unless a qualifying condition (terminal condition, permanent unconsciousness, incurable or irreversible condition) exists.*"

I turned back to my sister. "Maybe I should be the primary, since I've been handling all of the business stuff, and you're the secondary?"

The social worker interjected. "There's no place for a secondary. Only one."

"Well," Keith said. "I mean that's kind of true. Amanda wouldn't decide anything without talking with both of us."

"Of course not," I said.

"But she's at work during the day," Jackie said. "I'm the oldest. It should be me."

"I'll call you right away if there's any decision to be made," I said. "Besides, I'm handling the paperwork and trying to get the financials worked out. This will allow me do that. Do you want to take care of all of that? I mean you can take over the paperwork and finances if that's what you want to do."

"Finances aren't my thing," she said. "That's more you and Keith."

"And I'm pretty much unavailable," Keith said.

"So." I paused. "Should it be me?"

"Fine," she said to the social worker, "put Amanda down."

Jackie glared up at me and I looked away.

CHAPTER FIFTEEN

Meltdown

AFTER THE STAFF left at five, Jackie and I returned to the hospital to visit Dad. We gave the nurses the cupcakes and they cheerfully updated us on his condition. They told us not to mind the visiting hours and that we could stay as long as we needed to. Jackie winked at me.

Within minutes of getting into his room—luckily, he still had a private room—I was assigned the task of feeding him his dinner bedside while Jackie sat by the window. The nurses wanted Dad to feed himself but he refused. I pulled the table with the meal tray closer to me and twirled some short strands of spaghetti onto a fork. Dad opened his mouth. It reminded me of the 'here comes the airplane' game when my boys were babies.

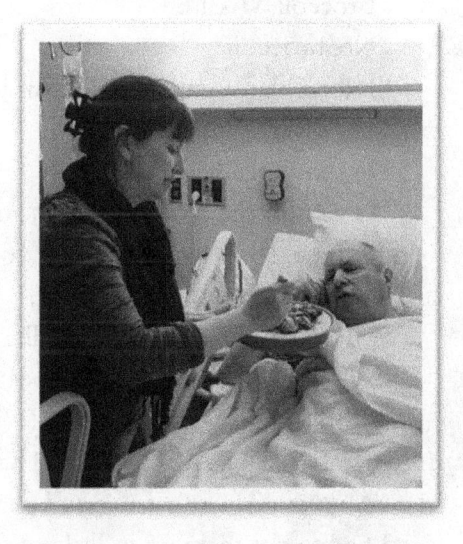

Justin was a fussy baby. Oh, as a young, new mom, how often I wished to have the support of my family. Often envious of my friends whose parents helped out, even if only a couple times a month, I was painfully aware of my dad's absence. Neither of my boys had a grandpa. No one to swing them in the air, sneak them cookies, play games with them. Because my mom was also too busy to help much, I made do without parental reassurance that I was on the right track, without having someone on the other line of the phone to answer my panicked parenting questions. Instead, I navigated it alone. Without my dad, Justin's grandpa.

And when David was born, my dad wasn't there to greet him into this world. It would be one thing if he were dead, but it was altogether another feeling to know mental illness was keeping us separated. He missed all of those baby phases, things grandparents who were good parents deserved to be ab le to enjoy. I doubted Dad had any concept at all of what he'd missed out on in his grandchildren's lives. All of the firsts—first steps, first words, holidays, birthdays.

I fed my dad another bite of pasta and wiped the red sauce from his chin. I imagined he had done the same thing with me over forty years ago.

There was a gorgeous view of Lake Michigan in the waning sunlight visible through the room length wide window. When Jackie turned towards me, I realized she was filming us with her phone again.

"What else is there?" Dad asked while I spoon fed him more pasta.

"Broccoli," I said.

"No, broccoli."

"I don't blame you." I poked around on the plate. "There's also a chunk of cauliflower."

He shook his head.

"Give him the apple juice." Jackie handed me a Styrofoam cup with a bendy straw. "Boy, look how neat you are, sis. You haven't made a mess at all."

I shrugged. "Giving him smaller bites."

"What else is there?" Dad repeated.

"More apple juice," Jackie said. "I told them to bring you extra because I remember it's your favorite. That was always your favorite, do you remember that? Here's water and peaches. Amanda, give him the peaches."

I had to cut them up in little pieces while she teased me for doing so.

While the feeding session continued, she and I unloaded the last ten years of stories of his grandkids—the two youngest of whom he'd never met—David and Jackie's youngest daughter. When Jackie and I last visited

Dad in Chicago in July 2006 before his disappearance, Jackie's oldest daughter was only three; Justin was only nine.

Dad didn't say much even when he wasn't chewing food. But he seemed to be listening and watching us, even if he wasn't talking.

Even if given the chance, Jackie doubted she'd want to subject her daughters to meeting this stranger, even if he technically was their grandpa. I didn't have the same misgivings. My boys, much like me, weren't ruled by emotions, which is why I'd often been accused by her of not having any.

Visiting hours were over, and even though we figured we could get them to make an exception, Jackie and I were exhausted. We hadn't slept well in days, since before the call came through on Monday.

We each gave Dad a hug goodbye. Even though we'd see him again in the morning, both she and I held the embrace as long as he would endure. This was nothing like leaving a loved one who you had the luxury of taking for granted that you'd see every so often—no, this was nothing like that. It was hugging someone you thought you'd never see again—someone you didn't know if you ever would see again. Yet, someone you had already lost.

Tony couldn't have given us a warmer welcome. When I stepped into his apartment, the first thing I laid eyes on was a console table hosting a candy bar—a multitude of glass jars and containers filled with confectionery sweets—*Reese's Pieces, Red Vines*, chocolates and miniature candy bars. What a welcome sight.

"I didn't know which deep-dish pizza you liked best, so I ordered from two places." He presented the kitchen counter taken up by two boxes of warm gooey goodness.

We sat around his kitchen table in a small dining room that looked more like a worshiping room for the Chicago Cubs baseball team. All available space in a curio cabinet and shelves were occupied by blue, red, and white Cubs memorabilia. I had forgotten how serious the fans were—win or lose—about their team. The other wall decor revolved around *Star Wars* while his living room mantle was an alter to *Seinfeld*.

"I have to go to work in the morning." Tony turned to Jackie. "And knowing you, you'll still be asleep. Amanda, you can sleep in the second room. Jackie, you can have my bed. I'll sleep on the couch."

"You don't have to do that," she said.

"Yes, I do. It's not often that I get to see you."

"Yeah, well, it could've been in better circumstances."

"I'll take what I can get."

I excused myself to get ready for bed while the two of them caught up for lost time.

Tomorrow would be the day Dad would be transported back to his facility. It would be the last time we'd be able to visit before leaving, therefore, the only day to convince him to sign the Surrogate Decision-Making Form. I drifted off to sleep hoping things would go smoothly, as they hardly ever seemed to do.

In the morning, I got dressed, but my sister dilly dallied. She seemed to be in no rush.

"Are you almost ready?" I prodded gently, not wanting to provoke her. "We need to go."

"What's the rush?"

"I don't want to run out of time."

"Stop stressing so much. Calm down. There's plenty of time."

I looked at my watch. After ten. It could be an hour's drive to the rehabilitation facility.

"How much longer?" I said. "I want to get there before lunch to talk with the staff."

She shut the bathroom door. I paced then sat on the couch, ate a slice of cold sausage pizza and glanced at my phone every few minutes. What was taking so damn long?

Finally, Jackie emerged and went back to the room to change. I kept my mouth shut.

Five minutes. Ten minutes. Come on, what, was she putting her jeans on with her teeth?

I heard sniffles, the kind that came with muffled cries. Dad's situation and seeing him again must have hit her hard today.

I remembered how, back when our grandparents were alive and had prepaid an apartment for Dad, I had spent a week with him traversing the streets of Chicago and New York—a memorable trip to say the least. And how, when he was homeless, I was able to get him off the streets of Atlanta and provide him with shelter for two months until I felt Justin was endangered by the unpredictability of his schizophrenic outbursts. And, all through the years, there were the sometimes-relentless phone calls, emails, and letters. And the months and years of waiting.

But that was my story. Hers was different. While Keith and I grew up with our mom and visited Dad every other weekend, Jackie lived with him pretty much every day of her life. She graduated college before Dad's mind turned on him after his successful cancer surgery.

After he roamed the world and came back penniless to live and preach on the streets in America, Jackie had only limited communication with him. She couldn't handle the emotional intensity of the rollercoaster of his illness. Since 1999, she'd only seen him once in 2006 in Chicago—while he resided in the prepaid apartment—then nothing until now.

Maybe I'd had more time to process the changes because I'd been a witness to it. And, taking after Dad, I had more of the emotional distance needed to deal with it all.

I crept down the hallway. Her door was cracked open. Jackie was dressed but sitting hunched over on the floor crying.

I entered, sat down beside her and placed a hand on her shoulder.

"Are you okay?" I glanced over her shoulder; there were photo frames and pictures in front of her, but none of them had Dad in them.

"I—I just…" Her sobbing made the sounds incomprehensible.

After a few minutes of cajoling her, she conveyed to me that the source of her sadness was related not to Dad, but to her relationship with her mom and two brothers and their family's lost time.

Perhaps I should've been more understanding, but heat rose to my cheeks. We were going to miss handling important business matters over her tears—tears that could wait. I swallowed hard and took a measured breath.

"I'm sorry you're having a hard time, but we need to go."

"Go? You don't understand." The tears took over again.

"No, you don't understand," I said, standing up and speaking as calmly as I could. "We need to go. We can talk later."

"You don't care about me. It's only about you and what you want."

"Are you fucking kidding me? This isn't about you. This isn't about them." I pointed to her family pictures. "We didn't fly across the country for this. It's about Dad. And if you don't want to come, fine. That's fine with me. But I'm leaving with or without you in five minutes."

Before she could swing at me, I turned and stomped out the door.

CHAPTER SIXTEEN

THE FIGHT

WITHIN FIFTEEN MINUTES, I reversed the car out of Tony's driveway while my sister sat in the passenger seat, silent with arms crossed. She focused her attention out the window; I focused on navigating the roads and highways to avoid the tollway.

Good. Maybe she would be quiet and we could get there without killing each other.

Wishful thinking.

Halfway there, with the back of her head towards me, she spoke. "You want to know what I really think?"

"Go for it." Whatever she said meant that whatever I said would be fair game in my mind. Overwhelmed and mentally, emotionally, and physically exhausted, the irritation was making me combative.

Over the next few minutes, while I accused her of being weak and selfish, she accused me of being arrogant and heartless. Increasingly personal and vindictive accusations and insults flew through our mouths ending with both of us crying big ugly, angry tears.

"Oh, my sis actually has feelings?" She rolled her eyes.

"Just because I don't cry all the time doesn't mean I don't care."

"Could've fooled me."

"You have no idea what I go through. I have to be strong to take care of everything. Or who else is going to do it?"

"No one's making you do anything."

"What have you done? You always make things worse. I wish you weren't here."

"You think you're better than me?" She burst out in sobs, screaming at me in between gasps for air. "Sorry for having feelings. Sorry for caring. Sorry for being here."

My stomach sank. I couldn't take it back. I didn't mean to be mean. But anger comes from hurt. "You don't appreciate anything I'm doing."

"Yes, I do." Her sobs continued. "I couldn't do what you do. I guess I'm good at nothing."

That wasn't true. It was her thoughtful suggestion that we stop by the store to pick up cookies and cupcakes for the staff. She was always thinking of these things whereas I focused on the forms and business end; so, in this way, we complemented each other and made a good team.

The stress of having a loved one, in our case, a parent, with a severe mental illness, an SMI, could bring out both the best and worst in a person, sometimes at the same time. If we siblings didn't kill each other over it, we'd do the best we could to offer what support we were currently capable of offering.

Keith wasn't there and neither of us could fault him for that, so we couldn't be bitter about that, either. Caring for a sick family member, missing or not, had a way of either dividing or bringing together a family. Sometimes it was hard to tell which way it'd go, how much to forgive, and when to let it go.

We both were emotionally drained and road the rest of the way in silence. I parked across the street from the rehabilitation center and turned to face her.

"Ready?" I asked.

She shrugged. "Thanks for driving. I probably would've gotten us lost."

I took a deep breath. "Sorry for being mean. Look, Dad needs both of us."

"You don't need me."

"Yes, I do. We're different but it would be more annoying if we were the same. Can you imagine two of me? We'd be robots."

She nodded. "Or two of me? A crying mess." She gave me half a smile. "I'm sorry, too."

I reached over and gave her a hug. She hugged me back.

"Jackie, the way you handled the social workers yesterday was great. I was getting so pissed at them."

"A gentle approach sometimes works better."

In the end, we agreed we loved each other even if we didn't always understand each other, both guilty of making assumptions about the other. We both grieved for Dad, albeit pain manifested differently in the two of us—she an open book, me a closed one.

We wiped our eyes (she cleared the mascara from under hers), and, arm-in-arm, we crossed the street.

We hadn't gone in the patient area before, so it wasn't until a nurse led us down the hallway to Dad's room that I really noticed the building's interior aesthetics, or lack thereof. The vinyl floorboards were discolored and peeling, and missing in other parts. The speckled linoleum flooring in the hallway was scuffed with grooves and chips. The walls may have been bright white at one time but now they were dreary, with zig-zagging gray marks running across them.

The faint odor of urine and dirty diapers permeated the space; it wasn't quite a stench but I could detect the essence of these scents in the air, like you'd do when perceiving hints of earthiness and notes of blackberry with a glass of fine wine. Although much grosser.

We passed a man in a hospital gown in a wheelchair stationed in the hallway who would occasionally roll his wheels a few feet then stop again. A woman moaned and wailed out from another room. Jackie and I stared straight ahead and focused on finding Dad.

A nurse brought us into a room on our right. His was the first of two beds, separated by a curtain pulled three-quarters of the way shut. I saw a quilted blanket on the foot of the bed nearest the window hidden behind curtains. Both sections of the room contained a small bedside table and a simple dresser with a small TV mounted over that—the kind of fake wooden furniture that would have been dated in the cheapest of roadside roach motels.

There Dad was, lying awake in the first bed. His head was nearly flat on the bed. I reached around to feel the lack of fluff in the plastic-coated pillow-esque thing covered with a coarse cloth pillowcase. The sheet and tattered blanket were askew by his feet.

He was dressed—thank goodness!—in a pair of dark gray sweats and a lighter gray sweatshirt, his arms raised above his shoulders making a goal post frame around his head, which raised his sweatshirt and exposed a thin strip of his belly. It looked quite uncomfortable. I pulled the shirt down slightly to cover the exposed skin in case he was cold.

Dad didn't let us turn on the bright light overhead. With the hallway and filtered room light, I realized his face had been shaven and his balding gray hair was closely shaven as well. He still wore a plastic hospital ID band on his left wrist—unless, of course, he was required to wear one in this facility—I didn't think it important to ask.

Although they told us Dad had been walking on his own accord prior to the recent heart attack, we found a walker and wheelchair next to his bed—just until he got his strength back, we were told.

Fortunately, Dad, although not very talkative, agreed to sign the surrogate forms for the social worker. We took a copy, just in case their copy became "lost."

Jackie and I competed for Dad's attention, both us racing to show him rolls of digital film. It was clear we hoped to get a reaction from showing him pictures of family memories—all of which he'd been absent from, plus family milestones he'd missed, and loved ones whose love he never had the opportunity to share.

"Here's me and my sons." I held my phone screen inches from his face.

"Amanda, let me show him the girls." She held up her phone. "Here, Dad, this is my daughter's fifteenth birthday, she'll be sixteen soon—"

"Dad, remember Justin? Look, he's twenty-two now. Can you believe that?"

"And here's Jim and me and the girls in Hawaii—"

"And this is David, your grandson who is eleven—

"And here's our house. It's beautiful up in northern California. Do you remember taking us on trips up there?"

"I took my boys on the road trips you took us on," I said. "I drove them up to Victoria Island in Vancouver, Canada. We had High Tea at the

Rose Garden in Butchart Gardens. Do you remember how we made fun of the name when we were there with you as kids?"

Dad didn't move. His lips didn't upturn in a smile. He didn't laugh. He just moved his eyes from one of us or our phone screens to the other then closed his eyes. There seemed to be a lot on his mind that he wasn't sharing.

"Are you tired, Dad?" I asked.

"You're not saying anything," Jackie said.

He gave the slightest shrug of his shoulders and opened his eyes. "I'm not much of a talker."

My sister and I laughed and said, "Since when?"

Growing up, my sister and I were trained in the art of verbosity from him. Hilda just listened and Keith never had the chance to get a word in edgewise. Dad could talk your ear off, even over the phone, and my sister and I took after him in this regard. Ever since we found Dad, the phone calls with him were one-sided with only his silence on the other end. He had changed; we had not.

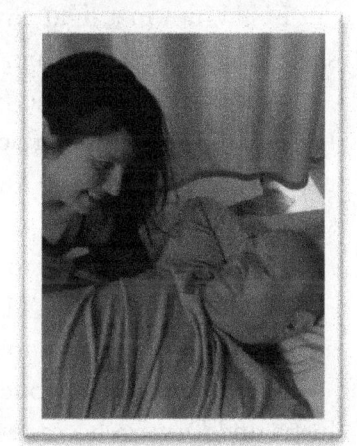

"We've got to head back to the airport soon," I whispered to her.

"Okay." She motioned with her eyes and held up her phone.

I understood she wanted to record footage of us with Dad for posterity. She filmed while I snuggled up alongside Dad on the edge of the twin bed. I rested my head on his shoulder. I hadn't done that since I was a child.

"Am I hurting you?" I asked.

He shook his head. "No." Every word seemed to take extra effort.

His reaction was neutral as I scrolled through my pictures and shared details of Justin and David and my dogs, one of whom resembled one of the two poodles Dad had so long ago. The ones who he used to take on walks and pet on the couch while watching TV. Also, the same ones he kicked down the stairs before he abandoned Hilda in a remote town in West Virginia when he hallucinated that they were all from the devil.

"Amanda, it's my turn," Jackie said.

"Wait, just a second. Let me show him a photo of Leo." I felt the minutes slipping by.

She threw me a look. Okay, best not to argue or fight over Dad in front of him.

I held him in a tight embrace, then stepped back to record her while she squeezed alongside him on the other side on the twin hospital bed.

I recorded her as she tried her best to engage him in conversation. Instead, she got grunts of acknowledgement while she flipped through her photos. Again, it seemed Dad's head was filled with thoughts he wouldn't share.

He yawned and blinked. That was our cue. Time to say goodbye.

"I talked to the staff," Jackie said. "They said they'd provide you with a chair so you don't have to stand in the hallway to talk on the phone."

I gave him a mostly one-sided hug. "I'll be back in a few months with Justin and David who can't wait to meet you. I'm going to take him to all the museums you showed us." I reached over for another hug. "I love you, Dad."

"I love you, too," he said, in the familiar flat voice, no intonation or animation.

Jackie leaned for her hug goodbye. "I love you, Dad."

"I love you, too," he said. Again, the words felt empty.

Neither Jackie, nor I, knew if that would be the last hug we'd ever give him.

CHAPTER SEVENTEEN
NAMI

I DIDN'T WANT us to miss our early morning flights, but I also didn't want to provoke my sister into an unwinnable fight. The sun wasn't close to rising. I hovered my finger over the button to order an Uber. She said she'd be ready by now, but she wasn't. In her defense, she hadn't been able to sleep at all the night before and had achieved Zombie status as she wandered around the apartment without focus.

Her brother helped us return the rental car last night, but we knew we'd have to get our own ride to the airport.

"Can I pack your bags for you?" I said.

She growled back, so I hid in the bathroom to wait it out.

Fortunately, no blood was drawn, and we made it to O'Hare Airport before the sun.

Before boarding two separate flights from adjacent gates—hers going to Northern California and mine to Southern—we said our goodbyes. Even though we'd found Dad physically, somehow it didn't ease the pain of losing him for so long. She had tears in her eyes.

"It's just so hard seeing him like that," she said.

"I know," I said, "but this is him now."

"He wasn't like this before."

"That was twenty years ago." I remembered she needed empathy, not my logical reasoning, so I reached out my arms for a hug. "You're right. It is sad."

Those thoughts swirled in my mind during my four-and-a-half-hour flight home. But we couldn't go backward, only forward.

Shortly after I returned home, I phoned Melody at the trust company to confirm we'd found Dad and that he was residing in a long-term care nursing facility. I told them I'd return to Chicago with my sons in mid-June. She was thrilled because it meant money could be sent to Dad for anything not covered through Medicaid.

Unfortunately, Dad progressively worsened after Jackie and I left. The nurses told us he was more depressed and paranoid. The voices were louder. Or maybe his mental illness had never improved; maybe the voices had never quieted—he just hidden it better while Jackie and I were there. Maybe that's what lay behind his vacant stares, him trying to shush the voices.

The staff were frustrated with him. He often refused his medication. The nurses couldn't coax him to get dressed, the physical therapists couldn't get him to put in any effort to improve mobility. He didn't seem to want to get better.

By mid-Spring, I sat on the couch with my sons, ready to buy plane tickets. Considering Dad's declining mental state, I second-guessed myself. Was it a good idea to subject my boys to him in his current condition? Would they be frightened?

I remembered when Dad scared me with his unstable and uncharacteristic temper, when I had to kick him out of my house for using and manipulating me and his parents while they were still alive. I hadn't felt safe around Dad then. I chose Justin's safety over my dad's well-being, because I couldn't do anything to fix him. As an adult, he legally could refuse treatment. And unless he was trying to murder himself or someone else, no one would help me to help him without his consent. But at that point, it would be too late. Catch-22. Discriminatory system.

But that was over fifteen years ago. He wasn't different, but I was.

When Dad disappeared after I last spoke to him in 2008, I educated myself on mental illness through a Family-to-Family educational and support class. That's how I found NAMI-OC, the Orange County, California affiliate of the National Alliance on Mental Illness, the largest grassroots organization focused on helping, educating, supporting, and advocating for those with mental illness and their families.

Back when Dad first developed a severe mental illness and someone had suggested I check out NAMI, I thought sardonically, *What can anyone teach me that I don't already know having experienced it?*

If only I had known what value there is in finding others who have or are going through the same thing. *You are not alone*, I learned, even if it felt like it from the sheer impotence of not being able to fix my dad, to save him. The brain is incredibly complex. I hope one day society finds a cure for severe mental illness.

After the class, I better understood mental illnesses and how they affect individuals and families.

This is why my heart ached in 2011 when Kelly Thomas, a 37-year-old man with schizophrenia, was beat to death by police. I read callous and ignorant comments from others placing blame on the family for leaving Kelly to live on the streets. As if the family had any choice. That hit me hard. It could've been my dad.

At the time, I still was helpless to locate Dad, so I turned that energy into advocacy for others. I spoke out at the County Board of Supervisors' meetings. I wrote letters to my congressional representatives. I penned letters published in the *LA Times, Orange County Register, and Sacramento Bee*. I passionately spoke to and educated others whenever I could to explain how mental illness impacts the entire family and how the system works against us. The healthcare system, the disability rights activists, the legal system, the courts—at times I've felt all of them were enemies. Roadblocks. By preventing loved ones, often the 24-hour caregivers, from being part of finding solutions, the system ends up harming the very individuals it claims to help. I learned about the revolving door of hospitalizations and jails, neither of which cure mental illness.

All of this is how I ended up on the Board of Directors for NAMI-OC in 2012, because damn it, if I couldn't save my dad and my family from the cruelty of the disease, I could at least focus my energy on helping others, to advocate for teens and for individuals living on the streets, for families and loved ones who need someone—anyone—on their side.

I wanted the world to understand, but often felt like I was shouting into the abyss.

When I discovered the Treatment Advocacy Center and met individuals who fight tirelessly to change the laws in every state, I realized that, yes, there are people out there who care, who understand, and who will not give up. I spent five years writing and researching my first book, *Losing Dad*, which was finally published in 2013.

I thought of the emails from readers who read *Losing Dad*. The teenager in Europe. The college students in Canada. The emails from across the country. The individuals at the NAMIWalk. The audience members at my speaking engagements. The ones who read the book and told me how it impacted them.

My story was not meant to entertain. It was written to help others understand how this is a societal problem. It was meant to provide hope, or at least comfort, to others who suffer. It was to tell the family's story, not to sensationalize the absurdity of extreme manifestations of the disease. To put our pain on the page, so that others can connect and make sense of their pain.

All of my efforts and energy devoted to the cause made this moment all the more surreal.

Yes, I had found him. But now what?

I stared back at my laptop screen. My sons sat alongside me on the couch watching TV. I had three round trip plane tickets to Chicago in my shopping cart. My finger hovered above the purchase button. I had a decision to make. Namely, do I bring my sons to meet a grandpa who may scare the shit out of them.

I remembered witnessing Dad screaming and cussing at passersby. If my sons saw this, would they be traumatized? Was I being a responsible mother to bring my sons around him, around other patients who shriek in terror at very real invisible monsters?

"Are you sure you both want to do this?" I said. "To meet grandpa?"

"Why wouldn't we?" David asked.

David—the boy who had participated at NAMIWalks since he was old enough to hold up signs. The one who told others he was walking for Grandpa, a grandpa whom he never met. The one who said his mom wrote a book that showed how mental illness impacts the entire family.

I nodded. "Justin?"

"As long as I don't have to share a bunk bed with him again." He smirked.

Okay, that settled that. I purchased the plane tickets.

"Do we get to see the German U-boat at the museum?" Justin asked.

"Yes," I said.

"And the coal mine?"

"Yes. In fact, why don't you and your brother plan the museums while I take care of the hotel reservations."

I stepped away and watched my sons sort through the exhibit choices. What were the odds of convincing Dad to come with us? These were, after all, his favorite museums, the ones he took me to when I was a child. But now he didn't seem to care about anything.

When I relayed my concerns over the phone to the nurses, they said we could check Dad out, like a library book, for the day if we could manage the wheelchair. But there were also bathroom considerations. Justin wasn't sold on the idea of helping someone who was more a stranger than a grandpa to him, in the bathroom. I figured we'd deal with that if we could get him to go.

I kept trying over the next couple months to convince Dad to come with us to the museums, or at least one. His answer was always no. Typically that's all he'd say on the phone, one-word or two-word answers.

Then, on June 1, his facility left me a voicemail. They had transferred Dad to the hospital the day before. "He was complaining of the chills, but when he got there, he was admitted for UTI and uncontrolled hypertension. Before he left, his blood pressure was very high, so that was the initial reason he was sent out."

Again? After having heart surgery only three months earlier? That being at least his third heart attack. I was angry with the universe. Why was this happening, again?

When I called the hospital, I spoke to a doctor.

"No, he's not having another heart attack," the doctor assured me. "But your dad seems depressed. He doesn't seem at all motivated to get better."

I couldn't understand it. He had to get better. We were flying out to see him in a little over two weeks. He had to meet his grandsons.

I thanked the doctor then explained the situation to my sons.

"We have to find a way to motivate him," I told them. "Talk to Grandpa about things you like. Let's get him excited for the trip." Excited? Well, I'd settle for pleased. Or even neutral.

I called the hospital back, put Dad on speakerphone, and turned to my boys. "Is there anything you wanted to tell Grandpa?"

"I like foxes," David said. He shrugged and mouthed: *I don't know what to say*.

"Yes, and he draws them," I said. "He's really good at drawing. Maybe he could bring a drawing for you. Justin?"

I pointed at Justin. Never the conversationalist, he glared back.

I gave him a pleading look.

He rolled his eyes. "There's the only German U-boat caught during World War II at the museum. They built a whole exhibit around it. Do you want to go see it?"

"Not really," Dad said.

"What if when we fly out there, we at least take you out to dinner?" I asked. "Anywhere you like."

"No."

"We can bring food to you. What do you want?"

"Nothing."

"How about barbecue?" I asked. "You always loved barbecued ribs." I needed to somehow motivate him lest he refuse to see us, or worse yet, decline in health or even die before we got there. "Remember when I was little, you took me to Chili's to get barbecued ribs?"

I turned back to my sons.

"Grandpa," David said. "Do you want us to bring you barbecue?"

"That would be okay."

Okay was better than no.

CHAPTER EIGHTEEN

THE NURSE

AFTER DAD was finally released back to his facility, the trust company suggested we hire an organization that specialized in eldercare to send a traveling nurse out to visit Dad. The nurse we hired would be able to monitor Dad's care. Because my siblings are I lived so far away, this sounded like a perfect solution.

I hadn't even known such a service existed. We were fortunate enough to have the funds in his special needs trust available to pay the hourly fees, which I figured was precisely the kind of thing my grandparents would have wanted for their only son who was all alone in Chicago.

We engaged their services and I spoke with Francine, the nurse who would be assigned his care. I suggested it best she didn't go until I could introduce her in person.

I could just imagine Dad screaming that she was there from the Mafia or CIA to murder him. Probably wouldn't make a good first impression.

"Don't worry," Francine said. "I'm used to visiting with patients who have a mental illness. I'll just stop by for a few minutes to introduce myself."

The first time, Dad refused to see Francine. Afterwards, I coaxed him over the phone to assure him that she wasn't there to kill him. He said it would be okay if she came back another time.

The next visit was successful, if you consider it successful that he didn't attack Francine.

"How did it go?" I said.

"I met with him briefly—"

"He actually agreed to meet with you?" Maybe she had magical powers.

"I sat with him for a while and asked a few questions, but mostly I was quiet."

"What did he say?"

"He was quiet for the most part. Finally, he told me my questions were stupid and when I asked, he told me I should leave."

"So, good progress?" I laughed.

"Actually, yes. I talked to the director of nursing and she reported that he is on his psych meds. The dosages seemed unusual to me but of course I am the new girl on the block and I don't know his med history."

"I'm shocked he's taking his medicine. Then maybe he's looking forward to our visit. Did he seem excited?"

"He struck me as quite depressed but staff tells me he's at his norm," she said. "I think it would be good to see if you can arrange to meet his psychiatrist when you're here."

"I don't know what to ask. Will you go with us? I'd like to meet you in person."

"Yes, of course, I can meet you there. And I can visit him as often as you want. Over time, hopefully he'll become more comfortable with me."

This meant, going forward, Dad would have a visitor every couple of weeks, a familiar face, something he hadn't had in nearly twenty years. The thought was bittersweet. I couldn't imagine not seeing family or friends for so long. How do you keep going when there's nothing to create, no one to see, nothing to look forward to?

No wonder Dad wasn't trying.

As our June travel date approached, I made one more call to Dad with my sons by my side. Was he still alive? Yes. Was he looking forward to our visit? Ambivalent.

"Are you sure we can't take you to the museums?" I said. "Those were your favorites."

"No."

"Not the Science and Industry one? The Field Museum? The Chicago Institute of Art?" I had fond memories exploring all three as a young child guided by him.

"No."

"Can we at least take you out to dinner?"

"No."

"Do you want us to bring you anything at all?"

"I want my Goddamn barbecue," he shouted.

My boys stared at me in disbelief. After I hung up, the boys burst out laughing.

"Make sure to bring Grandpa his Goddamn barbecue," David said.

"Yeah, don't forget the Goddamn barbecue," Justin repeated.

I shook my head and laughed right along with them. It felt good to find humor in the situation. So much of it wasn't funny. But, as I'd often heard, it's either laugh or cry.

I chose a thoughtful Father's Day card and my sons and I picked out cards for his birthday—Dad would be turning seventy-six in a few weeks. The boys picked out a small teddy bear as well—who can't appreciate snuggling a stuffed animal when you're all alone? We all agreed chocolate was also required in these circumstances, but we'd wait until we got to Chicago.

At least if we came with gifts, Dad would be willing to visit with us.

Maybe. As long as we remembered his Goddamned barbecue.

CHAPTER NINETEEN

POA

I ASKED FRANCINE to call or email me after each visit, because coordinating Dad's care from across the country wasn't easy. But according to Francine, her ability to help was tenuous. The staff was hesitant to share anything with her until I provided paperwork that she was there on the family's behalf.

"Is he taking his medicine?" I asked her.

"Sometimes," Francine said. "They said he does better when he's medication compliant. But I don't think he was during our last visit."

"Why do you say that? How do you know?"

"The voices seemed to be bothering him quite a bit. I encourage him to ignore them, but he's afraid his enemies are out to get him. And, he's worried they're after you."

"Great. That sucks. Can't we get him on an injection or something?"

"Agreed. It's terrifying for him. I would need to talk to the psychiatric nurse next time I'm there. But they won't speak to me."

"Why not? Dad already signed the surrogate form. I'm authorized to handle medical decisions and you're there representing me."

"No, a signed surrogate form isn't enough. They also need a signed medical Power of Attorney form."

"They refused to sign as witnesses on the POA document when I was there with Jackie."

"There's something else I wanted to ask you. Your dad needs some new clothes and he says he needs new shoes, too."

"Makes sense." I remembered the leather shoes and the nicer clothes he wore when I picked him up off the streets so many years earlier.

"We need to put his name on everything," Francine said, "otherwise, things have a way of walking away in a place like this."

"Sounds good. Is that something you could do, to get him some new clothes?"

"I could, but before I can purchase anything, you'll just need to make sure Melody can reimburse me."

I couldn't see why that would be a problem.

Apparently, it was.

When I phoned Melody, she explained. "Here's the situation. We're directed to spend the trust money for your dad, but now he's incapable of asking us directly. That means we need to be able to have you make the request, so we can approve it."

"Okay. I'm making the request. So, what's the issue?"

"It doesn't work like that. We need a Power of Attorney form filled out."

"But you didn't need that to hire Francine."

"That's a little different. We hired her. But in order to buy things for him, we need the form notarized."

"Can't you do that?"

Apparently not. We needed an attorney to draft the documents and a notary to be present.

"We can either hire an attorney," she said, "or you can get in touch with Laurie."

Laurie had been a lifesaver for my family. She and her husband had set up the trust for my grandparents before they died. If it weren't for the special needs trust, my dad and I would never have reconnected. It required partnership with the individuals at the trust company for me to locate him. The trust was how we were paying for Francine and could afford to help him in the future. Otherwise, Keith, Jackie, and I couldn't afford it. If there was an afterlife, his parents could rest easier at last.

"I'd like to meet you when I'm out there," I said to Melody. "Not just to discuss documents. But, after all you and everyone there has done for us—"

"Absolutely. We'd love to meet you. We're downtown in the financial district."

I needed to get the Power of Attorney documents as soon as possible. With the time difference and our busy schedules, I kept playing phone tag with Laurie. Then I became consumed with my Chicago trip plans and the documents slipped my mind.

The day before, I remembered again. This time I reached her.

"Yes," Laurie said. "Mike and I can prepare both the medical and financial property Power of Attorney forms."

"I hope he'll sign the docs," I said.

She paused. "I hope so, too."

The only other option was to go to court to get a conservatorship set up and I'd rather not have to go through that rabbit hole. It would be best if he'd willingly grant me the rights while we were still on good terms.

As long as the voices and his paranoia didn't get in the way.

CHAPTER TWENTY

Deep-Dish Pizza

On Tuesday, June 18, 2019, our plane touched down at O'Hare Airport in Chicago. This time around I reserved the rental car before getting there and the cost was more bearable at $220 for the four days. What a relief from the sticker shock Jackie and I faced back in February.

It was after 8:30 PM by the time we got on I-90 East. While we drove, Justin remarked on the last time I took him to Chicago, back in 2006, for a brief reunion with my dad before Dad up and disappeared for ten years.

"So, you didn't make us take the subway this time?" Justin smirked.

"It's called the L-train, and, no. Would you have preferred that? The Blue Line starts right at O'Hare. Remember?"

"Yeah, you mean when you made us drag all our luggage through the gates to get on? And then hold on to everything as it rocked on the train? Yeah, no."

I gave him a sheepish grin. "It wasn't that bad. Right?"

He glared at me.

"Okay," I said. "It wouldn't have been that bad if we had gotten off at the correct stop. I slightly miscalculated that one."

"Slightly? We had to walk for miles to get to the hotel, dragging our luggage on the sidewalks."

"It wasn't miles. Maybe a few extra blocks." I was never good at judging distance, so I suppose it could've been miles. "Anyways, we would've taken the L-train but we need a car to get around quickly, especially since we're staying near Miracle Mile and grandpa is up by Rogers Park. I told him maybe we could take him to breakfast in the morning."

After we checked into our hotel, I realized I hadn't fed my sons in half a day.

"Who wants pizza?" I asked. "I want you to try a special kind of Chicago Deep-Dish."

They groaned.

"I don't like that one," David said.

"How do you know? You haven't had it. It's made with cornmeal crust. You guys like cheese. Let's try the stuffed crust." I phoned in the order then turned back to my boys. "Good news is that the order is in. Bad news is that it's going to take over an hour."

I wanted them to appreciate the pizza, to create a warm moment between the three of us. I remembered being a young child, and again as an adult, with my dad ordering deep-dish pizza in Chicago. I had chosen the original place Dad had taken me to. But when our pizza finally got delivered, I realized the crust was bland and too dense. The cheese in the crust didn't add to it, but was chewy and detracted from the flavor. I thought back to sharing pizza with my dad—his joy and pride at ordering a pizza with the sausage patty that covered the entire surface, the sauce dolloped on top so as to not make the crust soggy, the Midwestern cornmeal texture.

And yet, this pizza in my adulthood didn't live up to the magical one from my childhood.

It's funny how sometimes we look at memories more fondly than they deserve.

David didn't finish his, but on seeing my disappointment, Justin went ahead and took a second slice.

Maybe it was never about the pizza. Either way, I was too exhausted to care.

CHAPTER TWENTY-ONE

Grandpa

WHAT DO YOU say to your eleven, almost twelve-year-old, son to prepare him to meet a grandpa he's never met who exhibits extreme paranoia and is delusional? The truth.

"Be prepared. If he yells at you or says anything mean, just know that it's the schizophrenia talking, not him."

"I understand," David said. "You've told me all this before."

"It's one thing to hear about it; it's another thing to experience it." And I hoped he wouldn't have to. I couldn't imagine being his age and being subjected to the confusion and discomfort that we as adults often feel around strangers on the streets with untreated SMIs who scream out at the world around and within. And to imagine that being your dad or grandpa… changes perspective.

An older woman with kindness in her eyes and smile lines on her face stood in front of the facility. She welcomed us when we approached.

"Amanda? I'm Francine." She opened her arms and I took her up on the offer for a hug. "So lovely to finally meet you."

"You, too." I introduced my sons. "I really appreciate you coming out this morning."

"I didn't want to interfere with your breakfast plans with your dad," Francine said.

"We didn't go." I shook my head. "He refuses to leave. Says he can't walk."

David and Justin glanced at the boisterous crowd of patients smoking on the enclosed patio, then back at me. I held up a finger to my lips for them to not say anything.

We entered the facility together and I smiled politely to the receptionist who buzzed us in.

While we waited at the beginning of the hallway to speak with a social worker and nurse, the boys peered around the corner and turned back wide-eyed.

"Where's Grandpa?" Justin lowered his voice. "I don't like it here."

"Mom, what's wrong with them?" David asked.

I stepped forward and rounded the corner. The fluorescent lights overhead painted a dreary picture. An old man in a hospital gown, partially open in the back, paced and spoke to himself. The faded scent of urine still permeated the air, covered partially by the smell of medicated creams.

I gave my sons a weak smile. "At least Grandpa is not on the streets. Here at least he has a bed."

Francine nodded and spoke in a whisper. My boys and I leaned in closer to hear her. "There are much nicer places. We'll try to get him moved to one. One step at a time."

Justin scrunched up his nose with a gagging motion like he wanted to hurl. "I can't. I need to get out of here."

"Relax. We won't stay too long today." Then to distract him, I added, "Where are the cards? Did everyone sign?"

Justin held out the blue envelopes.

A nurse and social worker appeared.

Francine and I discussed Dad's medication. I emphasized that they had the family's permission to talk directly with Francine because she was representing us in our absence.

"Don't forget we need the POA forms," the social worker said. "Also, you should talk to your dad about a DNR."

"DNR?" I wasn't familiar with the term.

"His wishes for his final care."

"He's not dying, is he?"

"No," Francine said and turned to me. "They need to know if he wants a feeding tube or comfort care, or if he prefers a do not resuscitate order. Trust me, it's better to discuss these things ahead of time."

The social worker and nurse agreed.

"Do you have a copy of the—"

She handed me the form before I could finish. Through the corner of my eye, I could tell Justin was barely holding down his breakfast.

"Where's the psychiatrist?" Francine asked.

"He won't be here today," the nurse said.

"I clearly spoke to someone the other day…" Francine took a slow breath. "Okay, what about the psychiatric nurse?"

"She's not here right now."

Obviously.

Francine turned to me. "Me being here for you isn't going to be very productive today, apparently. I'll say a quick hello to your dad and then leave you to visit." To the nurse and social worker, she said, "I will need to discuss his medications and dosages with the psychiatrist."

"Do you want us to show you to Joseph's room?" the social worker asked.

"No," Francine said. "That won't be necessary, thank you. I know the way."

With that, the two departed.

I took David's hand in mine and led him down the hall. Justin followed close behind. At last, we paused at Dad's open door.

"Your grandpa has a roommate," I said, "So we'll try not to be too loud."

"Could it be any louder?" Justin said under his breath.

"Joseph." Francine entered first. "Remember me?" He grunted. "Well, you have some really important visitors."

I stepped in. The boys lingered by the door, out of sight.

Dad had a short gray beard. Seated on the side of his bed, he wore sweats and a black t-shirt that advertised some illegible rock band. His furrowed brow, the frown lines drawn down his chin, slitted eyes barely open, lips pursed shut—his entire being resonated a deep sadness.

Francine excused herself and told me she'd be in touch.

I reached over and hugged Dad even though he didn't make much effort to hug me back. "It's good to see you again. Do you remember me?"

"Amanda," he said and nodded.

"That's right. I love you, Dad."

"Love you." Each word sounded like it took more effort than it should have.

"I brought your grandsons here to see you. Do you remember who?"

He nodded, again, and said, much to my surprise, "Justin and David."

That was the first time he'd ever said his grandson David's name. Maybe some small part of my dad, their grandpa, was still there.

I turned to my sons. "Come meet your grandpa."

Justin came first and hugged him. "Hi, Grandpa. Do you remember me?"

"He's much bigger now, right?" I said.

Dad nodded.

David entered next. "Hi, Grandpa. I'm David."

Dad nodded and said, "You like foxes."

How on earth did Dad remember that detail? The boys looked as stunned as I felt.

"Yes," David stepped forward with a grin and gave Dad a hug. "This is for you." He handed him a card. "And I drew you a picture of a fox."

"Here, Grandpa." Justin handed him the teddy bear.

"Thank you," Dad said, then sat there without saying anything else.

I wondered what thoughts were flying through his mind. Were the voices there? Was he sad at knowing how much of life he's missed out on? Sitting next to him were two boys who never had a grandfather in their life. Did Dad comprehend the depth of the moment? Could he?

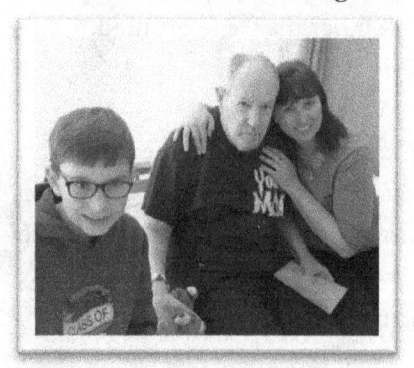

"Get together and smile." I held up my phone. "Closer. Smile." I snapped several photos then had

Justin take some of me, David, and Dad, with the teddy bear clutched in his hand.

While the boys chatted with him, which required prompting from me at times, Dad sat there and listened.

"Here, David," I said. "Can you take a picture of me and Justin with Grandpa?" I set down the cards and sat next to him. His mattress was thin, hard, and uncomfortable. I couldn't imagine sleeping on that every night. Then again, I suppose it was softer than a sidewalk.

"Okay, smile," David said.

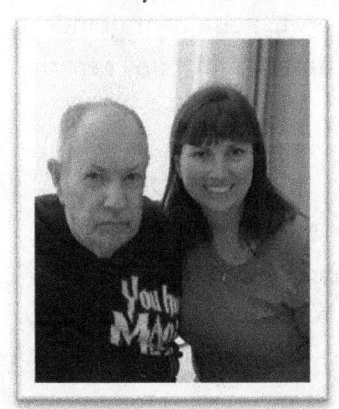

To my surprise, Dad wrapped his arms around me for the picture. Not a pull in tight embrace, but a simple powerful gesture just the same.

Still no smile from him, but I couldn't be happier.

"Justin, David, and I want to see if you need anything, so we can buy it and bring it to you in a few days. I remembered from last time that your pillow didn't seem so comfortable."

I squished the flat sad excuse for a pillow and peeked inside the rough pillow case to see a tan crinkled vinyl pillow covering. "Where are your clothes?"

Dad pointed to the tall cabinet. "There."

Justin and I opened it to find several empty hangers, a pair of gray sweat pants, and a random couple of t-shirts that looked like they were two sizes too big.

"Don't you have anything else?"

He shrugged. "They give me whatever."

"Mom," Justin whispered and nudged me. "Look at his shoes."

I went closer and realized the soles were separating and there were holes on top of the slipper shoes. "Dad, are these your only shoes?"

He nodded.

I remembered barely being a teenager and sitting in a Macy's Department store trying on black leather wedge sandals with my dad and stepmom Hilda. The sandals were much more expensive than any of the other clothing we usually bought. When I voiced my concern about the cost, Dad said, "It doesn't matter. Shoes are the most important thing. You've got to have good shoes." And from then on, I learned that to him, price wasn't a factor in shoe-shopping. We never bought according to name brands, but we did look for Italian and Brazilian leather. I learned to tell the difference between glued insoles and quality insoles stitched into the shoe.

Even when I first saw Dad after he'd been on the streets, he had on fine leather shoes.

And here he was wearing these ratty, torn up slipper shoes.

I told Justin and David to look around to see what else their grandpa needed. David held up a sad looking plastic toothbrush and a tiny generic hospital toothpaste.

"Do you have any floss?" I asked.

He shook his head.

Dad always had sensitive teeth and brushing and flossing were of the utmost importance to him. He made sure Keith and I did so every morning and night whenever we were with him. He paid for braces for Jackie, me, and Keith, bought us Oral-B toothbrushes with soft bristles, mint waxed floss, and Sensodyne toothpaste.

Back when I was in elementary school, I learned about the environment and the California drought and got into a passionate disagreement with him.

"Dad," I had pleaded to him. "Can't you please turn off the water while you're brushing your teeth?"

He shook his head and continued to brush.

"I'm serious. My teacher said we need to save the water." When he ignored me, I reached for the faucet to turn off the water. He smacked my fingers away.

After he spit out the toothpaste, he cupped his hand to scoop water to rinse out his mouth.

"Amanda," he said. "Don't listen to everything you hear. Brushing your teeth is not the biggest waste of water. If you're so concerned, take a shorter shower."

And he had a point.

"Grandpa," David said, disturbing my thoughts. "Do you have any socks?"

Dad pulled up his pants to show off the old pair of 1970s white tube socks he had on.

"We'll get you some new ones," I said. "I'm taking the boys to the museums this week. Are you sure we can't take you along to just one?"

"No, I can't walk."

I didn't know how true that was. "Well, is there anything I should show them?"

He rocked his head back and forth. "The coal mine."

I smiled. He remembered that. He took me there on our first family trip to Chicago over thirty years ago. It felt magical descending an elevator in the middle of the Museum of Science and Industry to go underground and ride in a miniature train to learn about the mining industry. It was on my to-do list for the next day.

"What are your favorite animals in the Field Museum?" I asked.

"The bears."

These were the most words I'd gotten out of him in a while. "And what should I show them at the Art Institute? That's where we're going today."

He shrugged.

"Do you remember showing me the house of miniatures?" When I was a young child, I held his hand while we toured the place.

He nodded.

I looked at the time. We were running behind to get to my meeting with Melody.

I stood up. "We need to get going, but we'll be back tomorrow."

"Don't bother." He lay back down on his bed.

"We came out here to visit you. We can take you out to dinner."

"I can't even shower without help."

"But you'll get better." I placed a hand on his. His skin was smooth and cold. "Remember you had heart surgery a few months ago. Recovery takes time."

He didn't say anything but instead closed his eyes, shutting us out.

"When we come tomorrow to take you to dinner, the boys and I can help walk you to the car. Or we can bring a wheelchair."

He shook his head, but opened his eyes. "I'm not going. Don't come back."

I dropped my shoulders. Why did he have to be so difficult?

"If you won't let us come see you tomorrow, would it be okay if we came back Friday? We flew all the way out here to see you every day."

"Fine."

I wanted to get out of there before he changed his mind. I motioned for the boys to leave.

"See you Friday, Grandpa." David gave him a hug then followed Justin to the doorway.

I said my goodbye and turned to leave.

Dad shouted, "Where's my barbecue?"

The boys stifled a laugh.

"No one serves ribs at nine in the morning. But I promise we'll find a place to get you some barbecue ribs Friday night."

"Did I hear you say barbecue?" A deep voice called out from the other side of the room curtain. A man slid open the curtain. "Are you looking for good barbecue, because I'll tell you the best place. I'll give you money if you get me some. Tired of the damn food round here."

Surprised, I introduced myself and my boys.

This man didn't seem like he belonged here—he was alert, coherent, and animated, but not in an emotionally disturbed way. He had a quilt and knitted blanket folded neatly at the foot of his bed.

"I'm just here in recovery," he said. "Be here a couple more days. Fell and broke my hip. Ain't that something. But hear, if I'm still around, you bring me back some. Best place, if you don't mind going downtown—"

"We're staying off Michigan Avenue," I said. "Not far from the Hancock tower."

"That's just perfect. Right there, that's the best place, if you don't mind the price, is Carson's. Now they got some ribs, let me tell you. My son brings 'em over sometimes. Just the best, I tell you. Real smoked meat. Not that wet stuff. The best. Been around a long time."

That settled that. Carson's it would be. I didn't realize it then, but the place owns the URL www.ribs.com. How had I not heard of the place?

When I perused their menu, I realized why. They were out of the price range of my childhood father, a former family guy feeding a family of five.

But you know what? Regardless of the cost, Dad deserved some good Goddamn barbecue.

CHAPTER TWENTY- TWO

The Collaboration

I FIGURED IT best to park the car at our hotel and walk or use public transit while we explored the city. But before I could take my sons to the art museum, we had our appointment at the trust company in the financial district near the river.

"Are we going to be late?" Justin asked.

"No." The time on my cell phone said, yes. One of my shortcomings: too optimistic about how much I could accomplish in the limited time I had. "We'll get an Uber." Besides, I wanted to conserve my energy for all the walking I knew we'd do later that day.

Once we got through traffic worsened by construction, we reached the address on Wacker Drive. I had to step out of the car before the top of the skyscraper came into view.

Security cleared us and we headed up to the 24th floor. While I had done an internship with a brokerage firm back in college, my sons had never been in such an affluent office before, marked with rich wood paneling and glass. They both were unusually quiet.

"You must be Amanda," a woman in a skirt suit greeted us. "I'm Melody." She held out her hand and a business card.

I shook it and glanced at the card which said Senior Trust Officer. "It's so great to finally meet you." I turned to my sons who were hiding behind me. "This is Justin and David, Joseph's only grandsons."

"Tell you what," she said. "I'll lead you to the conference room and if your sons would prefer to hang out in the waiting room, there's a TV and some snacks and water for them."

This perked them up.

I sat on one of the plush swivel chairs in the middle of the polished cherry wood table, long enough for at least twelve people.

Melody reappeared with an older woman with a pageboy haircut and glasses in a dark pantsuit. "This is Candace, one of our Vice Presidents. She helped set up your dad's accounts many years ago, when your grandparents were alive."

"It's my pleasure to meet you." Candace had a hearty grin and handed me her business card as well. "We're so glad you were able to make it here."

"Would you mind if some others join us?" Melody clasped her hands together. "Everyone here is so excited."

"Sure, sure." I nodded. "The more, the merrier."

Another few people joined us and introduced themselves as a Vice President and Senior Trust Officer, a Trust Administrator, and another assistant.

Everyone sat then the room came to a hush.

"Before we get down to business," I said. "Do you want to hear more of my dad's story?" It became clear from the affirmations around the table that that's why they were there, to hear firsthand the backstory of which they'd only half-witnessed, over the last fifteen years, to understand the man behind the illness and the illness that overtook the man.

I pulled out a copy of my book *Losing Dad* and slid it down to the end. "If you see on the cover, that's a photo of my dad." They oohed and aahed as they passed it around, flipping through the pages. "First, I have to thank all of you. Without us working together, my dad might still be missing, or even worse, dead on the streets."

They all leaned forward while I retold our family's story to my captivated audience. I spoke of the dad he was before, from road trips to folk dancing to hiking, to the beginning of the disease with the hospitalizations and suicide attempts, to the heartache and helplessness of his family during his international travels and subsequent disappearance, and the missing persons database.

"And so," I said, "Today was the first time he met his grandson, David. And he hadn't seen Justin in over ten years."

"That's an incredible story," Candace said. "I knew only bits and pieces. When your dad would come in to see us, sometimes I was here, but most times he just met with Melody."

Melody pursed her lips then let out a deep sigh. "I just can't believe that here you are, despite everything. I'm so sorry for what your family has gone through. I don't know how you've handled this. It's so unbelievable."

"Which is why I wrote a book about it."

Everyone laughed like a person who's experienced trauma but can find the dark humor in it afterward.

"Well." Candace uncapped a pen and flipped open a notepad. "Let's figure out how we can help."

We debated back and forth on the details of what Dad needed and how we could make it work. The basic facts didn't change—we needed Dad to sign the Medical and Property Power of Attorney forms.

"Laurie said she's emailing them to me,' I said, "so I'll bring them on Friday for Dad to sign."

"Good," Candace said. "As soon as we have a copy, tell us whatever he needs and we'll get the purchases approved."

"And what about Francine?"

"Yes," Melody said, "we will continue to pay for her services."

"And any medical bills and clothing?" I asked.

"Anything he needs, or wants, or whatever would make him more comfortable."

"I don't like the place where he's at," I said. "It's old and rundown and he doesn't seem to be getting the best care. He deserves better than that."

"Understood," Candace said. "We can arrange to have him moved."

"Do you know other places that take Medi-Medi?" Meaning Dad had both Medicare and Medicaid, the additional financial coverage for low-income individuals.

"We're not sure," Candace said, "but we can hire Medicare specialists who can help."

"Is he getting social security?" Melody asked.

"Yes," I said. "The checks are going directly to the facility. They had no information on him at all when he came in there. Nothing."

"Wow. We haven't heard from him in what..." Melody turned to Candace. "Has it been over three years?"

Candace shrugged. "It's been a good while."

"I need to find out how long he's been there," I said, "and see if I can track his whereabouts after he disappeared. I want to get a copy of all his medical records."

"Let us know if we can help in any way," Candace said. "If you need the trust to pay for an attorney, or whatever you need."

"There is one thing that's bothering me," I said. "My dad worked for seventeen years at Atlantic Richfield as a programmer and, according to Hilda, he's getting a small pension. Do you know where that's going?"

They shook their heads.

"I'm worried because the facility knows nothing about his pension, which means it's not going there. I didn't push because they started to ask questions, so I acted like I had no idea about anything. If they ask too many questions before I have answers... Well, I don't want to risk his placement there... What if they dump him back on the streets and he disappears again? We'll never find him."

"Is there a reason you're worried about the pension right now?" Candace redirected the conversation. "I mean of course, the money should go to the facility."

"Yeah, but here's the problem. Dad can't have more than two thousand dollars in assets according to Medicaid rules or he gets dropped. So where has all that money been going? I know he took it early, but even if he's only getting five hundred a month, and you said it's been three years, at least on your end, that could easily be over ten thousand dollars at this point. Maybe someone's been stealing his money."

A silence hit the room again.

"Did Dad always come into the office here to get money?"

"Initially, yes," Candace said. "But eventually, we set up a monthly auto transfer to his account. When we didn't hear from him anymore, we stopped the transfers."

"To an account?" I asked. "Which bank?"

"Citibank," Melody said.

"Great, what if his pension is sitting in a Citibank account somewhere? You know what that means?" I paused. "Medicaid finds out, they drop him, we don't have enough money to pay for the place, and he's back on the streets."

Everyone broke out in chatter about how no one would allow that.

"If it's only ten thousand…" The other Vice President spoke up. "I'm sure you can private-pay and in one month, that would be gone. You'd be fine."

"I hate to say it, but things haven't exactly always worked out for us."

"Things will be different going forward," Candace said. "We're working together now."

"I hope so. After I get Dad to sign the POA docs this week, hopefully I can get his company to send the facility his pension, and I can get info from Citibank."

Nods of agreement around the room.

"If for some reason…" I said. "If we can't get the POAs signed this week, my dad's shoes have holes in them and he needs clothes."

"We'll take that up with the discretionary committee today," Candace said.

"Thank you. All of you." I looked at my watch. "I better get going. I promised the boys I'd get them over to a museum today." I pointed at the book on the table. "Would any of you like to keep a copy of the book?"

Both Candace and Melody spoke at the same time, before Melody deferred to Candace.

I reached into my bag and pulled out another copy. "I brought a second one. Would you like me to sign them?"

"If you don't mind, I'd love that," Melody said.

"It's the least I can do," I said. "You helped me find Dad."

On the way down the elevator, Justin and David complained they were hungry.

"Why didn't you eat any of the snacks?" I asked.

They didn't want to impose and weren't sure how long they'd be there. Then they reiterated how important it was that we buy grandpa new clothing and shoes.

I wanted to hug them both for their thoughtfulness. My old dad would've been so proud of them.

CHAPTER TWENTY- THREE

FIREWORKS

We scrolled through online listings of local restaurants. I wanted to expose my kids to some great Chicago hot dogs. When I was little, my dad brought me to a place where I custom ordered the toppings on my dog much like I'd do at a sandwich shop. That's when I learned from him the faux pas of adding ketchup instead of mustard and pickles. To me, it didn't make much of a difference and I stuck with my ketchup and sweet pickle relish.

The closest place was Porto's. Just stepping inside was like walking through a Disney decorated version of an old circus or carnival.

"This is the place where you can order a cake shake," I said.

Justin and David eyed me expectantly for an explanation.

"They use actual chocolate cake and blend it up into a milkshake."

"Yep," Justin said. "I'm getting that."

While I watched them eat their hot dogs and share the chocolate cake shake, I realized that to them this was just lunch, not a memory to look back on. Then again, maybe that's how I felt at their age.

It seems it's only over time that we realize the significance of the mundane.

"Keep up," I said to my boys who meandered a few paces behind me, much like my dad used to say to me. "I want to show you Millenium Park."

"How much further?" Justin asked.

"Yeah, I thought you said we were going to the art museum," David said.

"We are. It's on the way." Their whining reminded me of my own at their age.

After we crossed Michigan Avenue, I paused in front of the Millenium Monument and convinced them to take a picture with me. It was there on that concrete wall that I sat next to Dad, Jackie, and Keith to take a photo in the summer of 2006. That was the last time Keith and Dad spoke. It wasn't a fight that got in the way, but a long history of injustice and misunderstandings. I wished Keith would talk to Dad. But, even if he did, what would they say?

We passed the silver metal bean statue. The boys stared in awe at the tall dueling pictures of faces that spit water at each other, the art installation known as the Crown Fountain, while I was happy to get a chance to sit on a bench and relax for a few moments.

When we got going again, at long last, the majestic green patina of the bronze lions came into view, the protectors of the museum stairs. This, too, held many feelings for me. I had taken photos next to them over thirty years earlier with Dad, Hilda, and Keith.

Justin and David tugged me to go in, but I paused a bit to admire the significance. Much like the road trips I recreated for my sons, this too, was a recreation of my childhood.

I hoped that my sons would look back and cherish this place as much as I had. But I know we're not the same. Neither of my siblings were as sentimental. I felt it my duty to safeguard and carry forward what had been left behind in the past.

My first goal as soon as we entered was to lead Justin and David downstairs to show them the Thorne Miniature Rooms. And indeed, as had I at their age, they found joy observing the artful craftsmanship of the many intricate details of the miniatures, the tiny dovetail construction of the dresser drawers, the painted cornices, colorful woven rugs, the hand-painted vases with colorful flower arrangements, intricately designed sofas and grand tables, each of them shrunk down to the size of a child's dollhouse.

I wondered if this is how my dad felt as he led me through these corridors, pointing out the rooms emulating the styles of different countries and eras. I felt proud to offer my sons the same experience. I only wished Dad could be there beside me, to reap the generational benefit of his parenting, to be able to enjoy his grandchildren. He deserved this, but the disease in his brain had stolen it from him and from me and from them.

While Justin led us through the knights of armor exhibits and the room of paper weights, I kept track of the time. I'd learned the importance of planning from my dad.

Back in 2006, Dad led Keith and Abe, Jackie and her family, and me and my family down to Navy Pier to see the spectacular fireworks. As was true back then, the fireworks display was only held on Wednesdays and Saturdays.

Because Justin, David, and I had to leave Chicago on Saturday, that evening was our only opportunity. But after we left the museum, we were greeted by darkening gray skies.

"Mom," Justin said. "I don't think there's going to be fireworks tonight."

"It's early. It'll probably clear up by then. Let's walk over."

"Walk?" He stood still. "It's too far."

"No, it's not. We already walked further than that today."

"Exactly. I'm tired."

"Let's go." I motioned for them to follow me. But it took me asking them three times before they moved their feet.

We passed through Grant's Park and the sky got darker and their moans got louder.

"It looks like it's going to rain," David said.

"Not necessarily. The fireworks aren't until after nine."

Justin pointed to his phone. "It's going to rain. The fireworks are going to be canceled."

"You don't know that yet. Besides, we'll get something to eat there. And I want to take you both to the Build-a-Bear store."

"Why?" Justin stopped. "I don't want one. Don't you think I'm a little old for that?"

"No, I made one with Grandpa only fifteen years ago. You can even get little outfits for them. I got a Cubs—"

"I know," David said. "You gave it to me. I don't want another one."

"Well, but there are other things I want to show you both."

"Can't we get a ride over there?" David complained. "My feet hurt."

"Or take the bus?" Justin asked.

"It's not far to Navy Pier. We're already in Millenium Park. Let's walk."

They groaned. The skies overhead were now announcing an impending storm. I looked down at my phone—the battery was at two percent.

"Mom," David said, "please, you're killing me. Plus, it's going to rain."

"It's not much further." Despite my fatigue, I quickened my pace. "Besides, my phone's almost dead. I can't order a ride right now."

By the time we turned down the road to Navy Pier, the rain came down, lightly at first, but steadily increasing. David tugged at my elbow.

"You have hoodies on," I said. "It's just a little water."

I looked past the dejected look on David's face.

The boys hurried to keep pace at my heels. If we could get to the covering of the building before the rain came down harder, we'd be fine. We could get something to eat there then head back to the hotel.

"I can order the ride," Justin said. "I have five percent battery left."

I glanced at my phone and powered it on. "I've got one percent battery but no signal. These skyscrapers aren't helping. We're almost there."

"My feet hurt," David said. "You're not being fair."

And that's when it hit me. I wasn't being fair. Not only that, but I was ignoring how exhausted I felt, too. I had compartmentalized my own physical limitations and allowed my brain to take over to achieve the items on our to do list.

I was, as my sister would accuse, thinking, not feeling.

I was doing the same thing to them that my dad had done several times to me and I hadn't liked it either. When Dad had made up his mind to take me somewhere, no matter how hungry or tired I was, he adamantly refused to change his course of action.

This had happened in Chicago when he wanted me to meet his Polish Barber, and in New York City when he hopped on a bus without me and almost left me to fend for myself across the street from the United Nations Building.

He didn't take my feelings or needs into consideration—I was merely along for the ride.

Maybe I was *just like Dad* as my siblings often accused.

But I had a choice. I did not have to repeat his mistakes.

I stopped and turned around. David was limping. Justin's hair was soaking wet, rain dripped down the scowl on his face.

"Okay, we'll get a ride if you can get a signal," I said.

"Let's go," David shouted.

Within seconds, Justin said, "Ride's on the way. We need to get up to that turnabout."

Thunder roared. The rain came harder and faster. I grabbed David's hand and we all jogged to the pickup location dodging puddles.

I shouldn't have pushed my sons so hard. And for what?

Things hadn't gone according to plan. But it's okay to adjust plans, to take other people's needs into consideration.

We had missed the fireworks.

Or was it only me who missed them? Come to think of it, did I even care that much about seeing fireworks? Or had I been trying to relive the memories I had with my dad?

CHAPTER TWENTY-FOUR

FINDING DAD

MY TRIP TO Chicago had been two-fold: introduce the boys to my dad and coordinate Dad's care, both financially and medically; and to introduce my boys to the beauty and culture of Chicago, the place my dad jokingly referred to as the farmer's New York City because of its Midwest roots.

On Thursday, after exploring the Museum of Science and Industry, I took Justin and David up the Hancock Tower, over a thousand feet above the ground. At the top, as the building swayed, I realized how my boys, much like my dad, were uncomfortable with heights. I remembered exiting the elevator at the top of the Sears Tower in the early 1980s, and asking my dad why he wouldn't come closer to the windows. He shook his head and remained in the center with his back pressed up against the wall until the time came for us to descend. That experience was repeated with him in 2004.

When I lay in bed that night, I felt a bit sad that Dad hadn't wanted us to visit today.

Then I thought back to my childhood road trip with my family up to Vancouver. Amidst the beauty of tall forest trees, we stopped to experience crossing an impressively long pedestrian bridge. Hilda and Keith proceeded across. Rather than experience the thrill, I stayed back to hold my dad's hand, encouraging him to keep going. We didn't get more than twenty feet beyond the drop-off when I couldn't coax him any further. I helped him release his death grip on the steel handrails and led him back to safe ground. So, even back then, we looked out for each other and I felt a responsibility for Dad's well-being. Some things hadn't changed.

I opened my phone and checked my Facebook messages. Earlier I had sent Hilda a few photos of Dad with me and the boys.

It was increasingly difficult to stay in contact with her. Hilda wasn't the most tech savvy and ended up with multiple Facebook profiles every time she either got a new phone or forgot how to login. And other times, I'd send her half a dozen messages over several weeks before getting a response, so that I couldn't be sure if the data was even getting through to her. Either way, it was frustrating.

But at least she had gotten the pictures of Dad. Hilda responded:

> Hello dear Amanda & kids, how are you? How was your trip to Chicago, did you a good time with grandpa? He looks better than the other picture after the surgery, that was nice of you Amandy, how was his reaction? How long you been there, I can't talk with you, because I'm in the house by the beach, no internet, & is getting cold, next week, I'll be in the city, I love you all. God Bless You, enjoy your vacation, bye-bye.

I messaged her a few more photos, turned off the phone, and tried to sleep.

By the time Friday rolled around, I checked my email for the umpteenth time hoping to find the POA documents in my inbox. But each time I refreshed my screen, they weren't there. I had hoped to print them from the hotel before leaving for the day so as to bring them by in the afternoon for Dad to sign.

So as soon as we entered the Field Museum, I left a voicemail message for Laurie.

Justin, David, and I explored the dinosaur exhibits while I kept refreshing the email app on my phone. My cell reception was spotty at best.

An email came through from Melody in response to my request to buy Dad shoes and clothing and other items:

> I took the request to the discretionary committee. We can do one of two things. You can purchase some shoes and clothes and send me the receipts and I will reimburse you from the trust or we can ask Francine to purchase the items if you do not have the time while you are here.
>
> Did you reach out to your father's cousin about doing a POA?

I slipped it back in my pocket and focused on my sons.

The Field Museum always held a special place in my dad's heart. He used to proudly parade me past the dioramas of preserved animals in what were portrayed as their natural habitats.

Dad used to love to point out the different species and read the information placards to me: Here are the black bears and their climate and diet. Here are the brown bears and their climate and diet.

I paced the corridors that wound through the mammals and birds, halfheartedly pointing out details to my sons. My dad would've done a much better job playing museum docent. I was too tired to put in much effort. I checked my phone again and refreshed the mail app. A message came through from Laurie's husband:

> Hope all is well with you. Please print the two attachments and call Laurie at your earliest convenience.

We couldn't have been luckier as a family to have had Laurie, my grandma's cousin, and Laurie's husband—both local attorneys. She was the same age as my dad. When she orchestrated my grandparents' trust, she had single-handedly kept resources available to my dad that he otherwise would have burned through in a matter of months. Quite literally, that may have kept him alive over the years.

"Mom." David poked me. "Justin and I want to go upstairs to see the gems."

"Not yet. I want to see them, too." I sat down on a bench. I was exhausted from standing and walking all week so the break was appreciated. "I just got a really important email and I need to read something."

He groaned.

"Do you want to go look at the T-rex Sue again?"

"We already did that."

"Justin," I called out. "Take your brother over to see all the foxes. There's a whole section of animal dioramas you both haven't seen yet."

They rolled their eyes but quickly became immersed in a corridor of wilderness scenes.

I scrolled through both State of Illinois POA docs until I got to the signature pages. Great. The medical one needed a witness. That's okay. Justin was twenty-two; he could sign as the witness.

The property one needed a notary. Awesome. There goes my hope of quickly resolving any issues with his work pension or accessing his Citibank account.

My phone rang. It was Laurie. Aware of the impropriety of cell phone usage, I cupped my mouth while speaking above a whisper.

"My husband and I are done preparing the POA docs," Laurie said.

"They just came through." I thanked her profusely. "How much can we pay for you preparing them?"

"Oh, no, Amanda. You don't need to pay anything."

"But all the work you've put in—"

"I insist. Everyone in the family, I assure you, wants to see your dad taken care of."

"There does look like an issue."

"What's wrong?"

"I'll have Justin sign as a witness for the medical POA, but the financial one needs to be notarized."

"I know. But you shouldn't have Justin sign, either. My husband and I plan to go over there next week to visit your father. We'll take care of all the signatures then."

"Fantastic. I'll let him know you're coming. It'll be good for him to have more visitors. He's really depressed."

"I can imagine. Why don't you at least talk to your father about the documents, so he knows to expect us and see if he'll sign."

"What happens if he refuses to sign?"

"The court would have to declare him incompetent. Let's hope we don't need to go that route."

Before taking the boys to the gem exhibit, I responded to Melody's email:

> Unfortunately, I will not have time to get him those things. He also didn't want to see us yesterday so we didn't go. He wanted us to skip a day and see him today instead.
>
> I did speak with Laurie and she prepared all the documents for both the medical and financial power of attorney. She and her husband will try to go see him next week to get him to sign. I'm going to prep him today to see if I can convince him as to why this is a good idea. She said they can go the secondary route if he won't sign, of trying to show he is incompetent, if that is the case.

After we finished touring the museum, we stopped at a Fannie May chocolate shop to pick up a couple boxes for Dad, to our hotel to print the POA forms from the lobby, and to Carson's to order Dad's barbecue. While I wished I could fit in a nap, I knew there simply wasn't time.

Dad loved coleslaw and beans, so I added those to the order along with cornbread. Even though a short drive up to the facility, it felt longer with the smoky sweet aroma filling the car.

We arrived at his facility before five. I requested a private room for us to eat with him, and they agreed to allow us to use a private break room upstairs, but that someone would have to escort us there.

While the boys and I walked down to Dad's room to wait for a nurse to help us, I remembered Dad's roommate. I had forgotten to get him some barbecue, but I'd be willing to share my portion. But when we entered the room, the second bed was empty. *Did he die?* I thought, horrified.

I greeted Dad with a hug. "Where's your roommate?"

"Gone."

"Is he okay?"

"He checked out this morning." He turned to the boys. "Hi. You have the barbecue." His expression was the closest to a smile I'd seen. I wasn't sure whether it was because of his grandsons or the food, or, hopefully, both.

"We got you this." Justin presented the boxes of chocolate.

"That's nice." While his face didn't smile, Dad's eyes did widen, so I took that as a smile.

David found the teddy bear on the side table and handed it to him.

Dad squeezed the soft bear in his hand and listened while the boys described the miniatures in the art museum, the coal mine and U-boat submarine in the science museum, and all the animals in the natural history museum.

"Can we eat?" he said as soon as there was a pause.

Before I could respond, a male nurse appeared with a wheelchair. "They said you wanted to take Mr. Joseph upstairs for a visit?" He sniffed the air and glanced at the bags. "Mmm... barbecue. Is that Carson's? Oh, man, Mr. Joseph, you're in for some good food."

"These are my grandsons," Dad said as we all made our way down the hall towards the elevator.

I was floored. That was probably the first time he had ever uttered the words "these are my grandsons."

"Is that right?" The nurse pushed the button and held open the door for us.

"Yes, that's Justin." He pointed from one boy to the other. "And that's David. He likes foxes."

In any other family, in any other world, these few simple words would be expected, nothing out of the ordinary, hardly noticed at all. But in this moment, under these circumstances, these words were not only extraordinary but miraculous. I leaned back against the back of the elevator as Dad introduced the nurse to his grandsons.

My world, my entire world, changed in that moment.

That's when I knew, that despite everything the schizophrenia had stolen from us, the past twenty-three years, that I had finally, finally, found Dad. And not just a physical shell of the man, but a sliver of the real person he was, a tiny remnant of the grandfather my sons should have had.

I had long ago accepted that Dad would never be the same. He was gone, yes. But I had forever wondered if any of his heart and soul remained.

This moment was confirmation that yes, yes, he was still there.

CHAPTER TWENTY-FIVE

Missing Money

I DIVVIED UP the ribs, coleslaw, potato wedges, and cornbread. While Dad, David, and Justin ate, I took pictures and videos. I never could tell when it would be the last moment. I wanted to preserve memories for posterity.

"How's your ribs?"

"Fantastic." David said with his mouth full.

Justin nodded.

"Come on, eat." Dad motioned for me to put away the camera. I coerced him into a couple selfies before I complied.

And yes, the ribs were delicious. The wet wipes were pretty useless, but as soon as everyone cleaned up, I broached the subject of the POAs.

I explained both forms to him and he said he understood.

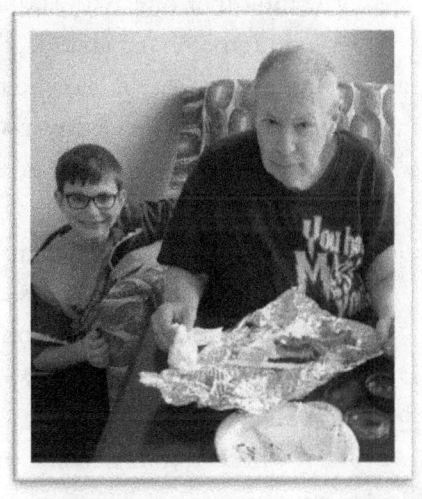

"So really, this medical one will enable me to make healthcare decisions for you, if you're unable to do so. That way I can make sure everyone respects your wishes." What were his wishes? I went through the DNR options with him. He selected comfort care.

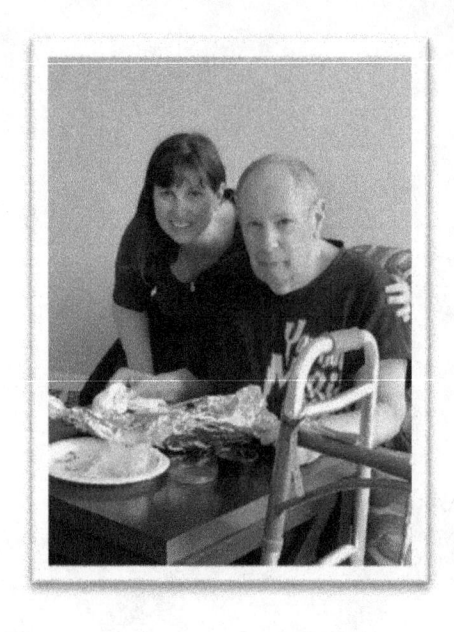

"I don't want any of that," he said when I mentioned feeding tubes.

"After you sign, I promise, no matter what, that I won't let anyone do that to you."

"I'll sign." And he did.

"We need a witness, so do you remember your cousins Laurie and Mike?"

He nodded.

"They're going to come by hopefully next week to notarize the forms."

"Why?"

"I don't want anyone to think you're not in your right mind. The nurses won't sign as witnesses, Justin can't sign, but we need to prove that you know what you're signing."

He rocked his head back and forth indicating he wasn't happy but understood.

"Why the other one?" he said, referring to the financial POA.

"Do you remember Francine, the lady who's been visiting you? She's a safe person for you to talk to. The trust company sent her to help you. But they need you to sign this form so I can authorize them to pay her and buy anything you need while you're here at this facility."

"They're already paying."

"For this place? No. They didn't know you were here. No one knew."

He sighed and closed his eyes.

"Plus, I need to track down your pension to help pay for your stay here. Do you remember your bank account information?"

"Don't have one."

"Then where is your pension going?"

He shrugged.

"The money should be coming here."

"I don't know."

"Besides, I want to buy you whatever you need. Is there anything at all you want, in addition to clothes and shoes? A nice recliner chair? A new TV? A webcam so we can video chat?"

He shook his head.

What if he was getting paranoid again? What if he accused me of stealing his money like he'd done back in 2002 when I had to kick him out of my house for manipulating my grandparents along with his unpredictable behavior and temper.

"Dad, do you trust me?"

He opened his eyes and nodded.

I couldn't ask for more than that.

CHAPTER TWENTY- SIX

THINGS OVERLOOKED

SATURDAY, JUNE 22. Our last day in Chicago. I wanted to see Dad one last time before our flight home, but it wouldn't be easy.

"Are we going to see grandpa now?" Justin asked. He was the only one dressed, packed, and ready to go. Then again, he was an anomaly in my family—the rare morning person.

"It's going to be tight, but yes." I slipped on my shoes, stood up, took a deep breath, and coughed. The week must have been wearing on me, because the exhaustion hit me hard that morning. "First, we're going to the zoo and the flower conservatory—"

"We don't care about flowers," David said and Justin scrunched his nose in confirmation.

"No, I need to show you something there… the sensitive plant." I had fond memories of this place with Dad, and my grandparents. "And the Lincoln Park Zoo has a Fennec Fox."

David's eyes lit up.

"And then we see Grandpa?" Justin asked.

"Yes."

"Are we getting him shoes? Remember the holes?"

"If we have time… I don't know… we have to return the car and get to the airport… our flight leaves at 7:30 PM."

"How do we have time to do anything then?" Justin paced. "Let's go."

We headed out to the Lincoln Park Zoo on a mission to find the Fennec Fox. The heat of the morning was really getting to me so we stopped to get some food and water.

"It's over there." Justin looked back at the map. "Let's go. We need to have enough time to see grandpa."

I kept up with them, but paused in the shade here and there and took more water. Then I sucked it up, and kept going.

Because David begged me to, I snapped several photos of the adorable creature curled up in a ball, with a fluffy tail wrapped around the body. Then the dizziness hit me.

I stumbled out of the exhibit and sat on the nearest shady bench.

"Mom," David said. "Are you okay?"

"It's just hot... and humid... a long week.... have Justin... get me water."

While the boys ran to get me water, I bowed my head between my knees which made me dizzier. I lay down on the bench and prayed I wouldn't faint. I considered whether this was heat exhaustion and if it was bad enough for me to seek medical attention.

On the one hand, it was our last day and we would be home just after midnight, Chicago time, 10 PM in California. Leo would pick us up from LAX and we'd be in bed before midnight.

On the other hand, I was responsible for driving these two boys around and needed us all to be safe. And I felt like I might pass out.

But was it bad enough to miss our flight?

I drank a lot of water and rested another fifteen minutes in the shade when the realization hit me. I recognized these symptoms, but I'd been ignoring them all week. In fact, come to think of it, I'd had this inexplicable exhaustion for a month.

I'd first noticed it during a Boy Scout backpacking trip David and I had taken a few weeks earlier. I mean I knew I wasn't in the best physical shape, but I had to stop constantly to take a break. Granted the rain turned to sleet turned to hail turned to snow unexpectedly, and we ended up snow camping after our hike, which was a memorable but miserable evening, but still.

I took a deep breath, felt lightheaded, and coughed. Yes, I definitely recognized these symptoms. I bet I had walking pneumonia. This would mark my fourth case of pneumonia, two viral and two bacterial cases.

I swear if I could predict my death—it would be pneumonia.

But if I was correct, this meant I'd done a backpacking trip in the snow with pneumonia and walked all across Chicago with it, so I deserved a damn medal.

I decided I wasn't going to die today. I'd just try to slow down, drink and eat well, and breathe. I phoned Leo and told him I would make an appointment to see my doctor on Monday. If it got worse, we agreed that I'd go to urgent care in the morning, or the ER later that night if needed.

Before we left, I needed to visit a certain plant again.

At the Lincoln Park Conservatory, I led them on the winding paths around the plants. The humidity was horrible and I felt like I couldn't breathe, so I took frequent breaks.

"Stop," I called out. The boys turned around. I squatted low and reached my finger to gently tap on a mini fern leaf.

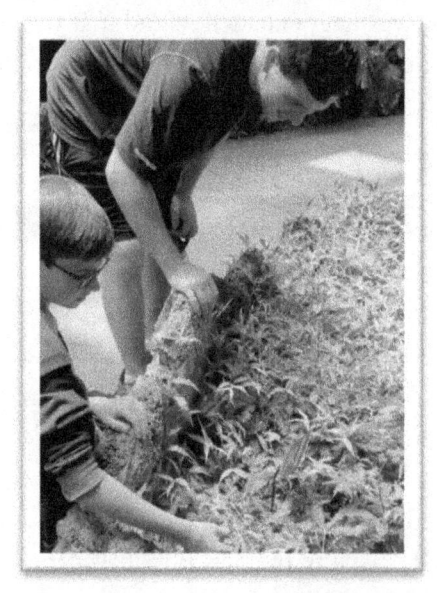

"Mom, are you supposed to touch it?" Justin whispered. I had taught them, look, but don't touch. He remembered well.

"Yes, look." I pointed to an arrow sign that said Touch. "It's a sensitive plant." They rolled their eyes. "No, for real. Look at the description. It says 'Sensitive Plant, *Mimosa pudica*, Leguminosae, Asia, West Africa.' Tap it gently and watch." I withdrew my finger and the fern leaf rolled up its delicate green sides.

Passerby stopped to stare at the spectacle they hadn't realized was important.

"It's so cool. It's like the plant has a mind of its own." David leaned closer. "Can I try?"

"Yes." I stepped back and sat on a bench to rest. "Your grandpa took me here a long time ago and showed it to me."

Back in 2004, Dad had fallen into a planter when I was visiting him in Chicago. He hadn't hurt anything except his pride. I had to go back to find his black glove and teased him until I laughed so hard I had tears in my eyes. He suppressed a smirk and smacked me back with his other glove. A moment of normalcy among the forest of insanity.

After the novelty of the sensitive plant wore off, the reality of my fatigue hit me again.

"Let's head back to the car, so we can see your grandpa."

"Before we leave, are we getting Grandpa clothes?" David asked. "I feel bad for him."

Justin turned to me. "The guy next to him had blankets. Can we get him one?"

I looked at the clock. Get to the gate on time, account for traffic, get gas, return the rental car, get back to the airport, get through security, so we could get on the plane to get home. 7:30 PM flight, be at the gate by 6:45 PM, minus at least one hour, minus fifteen, minus thirty, minus thirty, minus forty-five minutes to be safe. We had to plan to be out of there by 3:45 PM.

It was already close to two.

"Sure," I told them. "We've got plenty of time." Which of course we didn't.

CHAPTER TWENTY- SEVEN
Clothing

"We have to be fast." Still reeling from exhaustion, I leaned on the shopping cart. "Just throw everything in." Because of the time crunch, we sacrificed quality and ended up at Walmart. At least it had everything under one roof.

Polo shirts. Checkered pajama pants. Socks. Deodorant. Shoes? I remembered seeing the number eight on his ratty ones the other day.

"Grab a couple sizes of those slipper shoes," I said to the boys, feeling out of breath. "Size eight and eight-and-a-half."

After the fastest shopping trip that I'd ever been a part of, we had bags of clothes, a memory foam pillow, and a soft blanket. I relieved to be done with the standing and walking around.

We brought everything to Dad.

"I got this mattress topper for you," I said. "Your bed feels too hard."

"Grandpa," Justin said. "We also got you this soft blanket." He and David set it up.

"What do you think of the pillow?" I asked.

"It's too high."

"We can get you something thinner. Do you like the foam topper and the fuzzy blanket?"

"It's okay."

There wasn't a hint of enthusiasm in his voice or mannerisms—everything was flat.

"Can we show you the clothes?" I needed to rest, so I took a seat on the chair and motioned for my sons to display the items.

Dad shook his head, clearly unimpressed.

"You don't have clothes," I said. "Will you at least keep some of it?"

Out of the dozens of shirts, pants, and pajamas we had picked out for him, Dad only agreed to keep four shirts, one pajama bottom, along with the pillow, blanket, and topper. That's it. It was frustrating. No matter how much I understood that the mental illness was not within his control, still, it was frustrating to put so much effort into helping someone who not only didn't appreciate it or thank you for it, but didn't even accept it.

"Mom," David nudged me. "The shoes."

We had Dad try them on, but nothing fit. He indicated they were too tight and uncomfortable.

"Your shoes with the holes in them are probably a better brand," I told him. "And you don't remember where you got them. Next time Francine comes, she'll try to figure it out and get you a new pair."

"Okay." Another one-word response. I had gotten my hopes up the night before when he introduced his grandsons to the nurse. He had remembered their names. He even remembered that David liked foxes, but now we got nothing.

Justin pointed to the clock. It was 3:45 PM.

"Dad, we need to get to the airport."

He looked up at me and I saw a deep sadness in his blue eyes. Rather than find hope at seeing him display emotion, it hurt. Why, out of all emotions, did it have to be despair?

I reached in for a hug. "I love you, Dad. I will be back to visit."

He hugged me back. "I love you."

Justin and David took turns saying goodbye, and Dad hugged his grandsons and told them he loved them.

Those words hit me, especially in contrast to his sadness. Sure, he wasn't happy about the clothes. Why would he be when that's all he'd be left with after we departed? How it hurt to see him there in a strange place all by himself. To think of him being without family or friends for so many years was too painful of a thought for me to dwell on.

Focus on what's positive. We found him. He met his grandsons.

I ushered everyone into the car and headed back to the store.

"Where are you going?" Justin asked. "We're going to be late."

"What else am I going to do with the bags of clothes and shoes he's not keeping?" I pointed to the returns. "Help me. We have to hurry."

While we rushed to the airport, Justin stared out the window and shook his head. "Grandpa looks sad."

"I think that's totally understandable, right?" No need to sugarcoat it for them. "He realizes he's alone."

"That's sad." David looked at me in the rearview mirror.

Yes, of course it was. "Remember how he gave everyone hugs and said how much he loved us, right? That's a huge deal. Before your auntie and I visited him, he hadn't seen anyone he's related to in over ten years. And now he finally knows he's loved, so that's a special gift you both gave him by coming out to visit him."

"Are you moving Grandpa out to California?" Justin asked.

"No," I said. "He told me he doesn't want to leave Chicago. He likes the seasons out here."

David asked, "Why couldn't we stay here longer?"

"We have to get home. Besides my friend's birthday, Leo's birthday, your birthday, Uncle Keith's birthday, and one of my best-friend's weddings, there's a lot going on, not to mention I probably have pneumonia."

There was always a lot going on. Apparently for everyone, except Dad.

CHAPTER TWENTY-EIGHT

Mounting Problems

We got back in time. While Leo and I planned birthday celebrations and a weekend away to celebrate our fourth anniversary, I continued following up on the POAs and coordinating Dad's care. Reading and responding to the nonstop emails regarding Dad's medical care, finances, and future housing plans was like having a second job.

We all still had lives to lead, lives we made for ourselves in his absence, and lives that we needed to continue to live after I found Dad.

And as it turned out, yes, I did have walking pneumonia, and it was bad enough that it took multiple rounds of multiple drugs to get rid of. The doctor shook her head when I told her all the walking and hiking that I'd done while unknowingly sick. I was annoyed it had slowed me down.

Leo gave me a hug. "Babe, maybe it's a sign you need to take a break. You've been doing a lot. You've been so stressed out with your dad and everything." He kissed the top of my head.

I had to agree. The stress was too much. Having him to lean on at least made it bearable.

* * *

"I'll look for some shoes at Nordstrom Rack," Francine said. "Is there anything else I can get him?"

"In the past, everything I've bought him, whether it be clothing or furniture, he gave away to other people or decided not to keep."

"I'm sure he'll keep the shoes."

"I went through the few belongings he had there in a drawer. It seems he's thrown away every card and letter we've given him. He used to save these types of things." During my childhood, he had tall four-drawer filing cabinet and a meticulous filing system. Every folder labeled clearly and alphabetized. I'd followed in his footsteps with my own four-drawer filing cabinet, and had even gotten two-drawer filing cabinets for my sons.

"When the boys and I were out there," I continued, "he had a card from Jackie for Father's Day. He said he'd throw it away because he already read it, but I told him to save it so he could look at it again later. We also got him a card and a teddy bear. I don't know if he still has those."

"I'll check next time I'm there." Francine had a kind voice, the kind that made you feel heard. "I'll also let you know what the nurse says about his meds. I suspect some are off and may need to be adjusted."

A week after my return home, while I filed paperwork, I re-examined the items I had previously placed in the folder labeled "Dad." I spotted a huge problem. I immediately emailed the team at the trust company and relayed my concerns:

> I looked over the Surrogate Decision-Making form I have from the facility. It seems we will not be able to fill out the financial and medical power of attorney forms directly with my dad, because they had already declared him incapable of making decisions due to his "severe, persistent mental illness." Please see the attached form. What should our next course of action be in getting both documents completed?

Instead of replying back, Melody phoned. "If your dad is unable to execute powers of attorney," she said, "then the only other option is for someone to petition to be his guardian."

"But it doesn't make sense," I said. "He seemed quite lucid when we met with him a couple weeks ago. I don't understand where they draw the line on competency."

"When did you sign the form?"

"Back in February when I was first there with Jackie."

"Now that he's been medicated for a while, it may have changed. You need a doctor's note either way."

I sighed. "It's impossible to reach doctors there."

"I'll reach out to Francine and ask for her assistance."

So, this meant that the POA documents could not be signed lest we end up in court somehow. Petitioning to be a person's guardian was not a road I wanted to take except as a last resort. That could be costly and time-consuming, not to mention the horror stories I'd heard from others. The court can appoint someone to represent my dad who could potentially, in the guise of patient's rights advocacy, talk Dad out of agreeing to anything and instead encourage him to fight it. Granted, a person's rights need to be respected and nobody should be taken advantage of, but that would be counterproductive in our scenario. As is true for many other loving families experiencing this dilemma, it could mean someone isn't getting the help they need in the meantime.

While we were trying to sort through that complication, there was another, more immediate one to address: his medication.

Any family or loved ones who have gone through an experience similar to ours, knows how frustrating the medication roller coaster can be. And anytime a person is hospitalized or sent to another facility, the entire game changes. Suddenly the new doctors may act like they know best and, despite not understanding the patient's long medical history—which drugs work and which ones don't—they play Russian Roulette with the wheel of medicines.

This can destabilize a patient and undo years of fine-tuning treatment. Devastating is an understatement for how crippling this is to the family members who, without MD at the end of their names, are often denied any say in the matter. And even when provided with the medical history, it's often ignored. Not to mention that a new hospitalization or a different shift during a hospital stay means a new doctor. Why that's not medical malpractice, I can't figure out.

In my dad's case, I didn't feel like his medication had ever been fine-tuned. Besides which, a nurse informed me that Dad had been refusing his medication. For someone with paranoid schizophrenia, this meant the delusions and hallucinations, like fearing the mafia was coming after him, were probably worsening and becoming unbearable for him.

What little I did know of psychotropics was that certain ones such as Wellbutrin XL were not to be given at night. So, when I heard about it was being given at night and some other questionable dosing, I sat down at my desk with my notepad and my "Dad file," and contacted Francine.

"Can you confirm this information?" I asked. "Who can you talk to? It's like I can't ever get a straight answer out of anyone."

"Because the other nurse Jada was not able to answer my questions," Francine said, "I spoke with Stephanie, the Director of Nursing who was quite responsive."

"And?"

"According to her, your father has been on Wellbutrin for a while. It was increased to 150 mg every twelve hours in March."

I wrote the information down. "What about when he was in the hospital more recently?"

"She tells me the psych meds were continued in the hospital."

I shook my head. "That's a lie. While he was at the hospital, I spoke with at least four different nurses as well as with the doctor twice, all of whom said he was refusing all oral medications. That means there's no way he was taking the psych meds even if on paper it said he was supposed to."

"That's news to me. But I'm not surprised. I'm not sure how Buspar came into the conversation, but the first time I visited, Jada indicated he was on it when we met with her. In any event, it doesn't seem that he has been on Buspar."

"I don't know much about Buspar." I wrote it down. "But what's with the Wellbutrin at night?"

"I agree that an evening dose of it is very, very unusual."

"Then it's their fault he's not sleeping." Dad had been complaining to me about not being able to sleep.

"I would like to talk with the psych nurse practitioner to understand her thinking before making a judgment."

I calmed down knowing Francine knew more than I did about meds and was advocating on our behalf. I looked back over my notes where I'd written down questions about his mobility.

"Do you know why Dad is in a wheelchair?" I asked. "I thought he had physical therapy after the heart procedure, but when the boys and I were there, it was like he couldn't walk."

"He seemed to walk without problems, at least the short distance to the bed, where he sat up through our visit."

Had his mobility improved, or was it willful helplessness, like when he had Jackie and I spoon-feeding him in the hospital? "Is Dad finally talking to you when you visit?"

"He was much more easily engaged. He was very negative about the facility, but when I talked with him about alternatives, he wasn't interested. He told me that everyone he encountered was an asshole."

I laughed. "That's kind of funny." Some days I felt the same way.

"I asked him if he considered me as such as well and he said no."

"Well then, that's great progress. At least he enjoys your visits."

"He didn't remember my last visit."

"Why not?" The hair on my arm bristled. "He mentioned Alzheimer's a while back. Do you think he has it?"

"I'm not sure yet. He talked about his education and his work as a math teacher, but many things he stated, 'I can't remember.' I was careful not to ask too many questions. I told him how much I appreciated his willingness to talk with me. So, a little opening with him." She seemed to detect my concern and added, "Don't worry too much. I'll speak with his doctor about the memory."

I glanced down at the Walmart receipts from our last shopping trip for him. "What about the shoes?"

"The shoes I brought did not suit him. The ones he has are Merrell—practically indestructible, it seems. He didn't think he needed new ones as he doesn't go outside. But I'd like to see if we can get him out soon. I told him I'd bring new Merrell shoes and he could decide if he wants them."

Merrell shoes weren't cheap, so I imagined that if she could get the right size, he'd keep them.

We were so fortunate to have Francine helping our dad. Without her, would Dad's life have been better, seeing family members a couple times a year? At least we had the funds available to pay for her services. What about all the other families out there who couldn't afford it? Besides which, many people out there like my dad, because of their severe mental illness, are estranged from family and friends. I counted my blessings.

The next week, after the birthdays and wedding had come and gone, which provided a lovely distraction being around family and friends, I refocused my attention on both Dad's medicine and POAs.

I phoned Dad for his birthday.

"Happy birthday," I said, but didn't ask him how it was, because I already knew the answer. How fun could it be to celebrate your birthday alone in a nursing home?

"Thank you," he said.

"Did Francine visit you last week?" I wanted to see if he remembered.

"Yes."

"I think she brought you shoes."

"They didn't fit."

Happy to get an entire sentence out of him, I kept talking. "What about the new pillow we got you?"

"It's nice. But I'm still not sleeping well."

"I'm sorry. That's frustrating." I chose not to bring up the topic of medication; I'd let Francine handle that. "Did you get the Father's Day card I sent you?"

"Yes, it was nice. Thank you."

"Last time we were there, you were using the wheelchair. Are you still using it?"

"No, I'm getting better at walking." He cleared his throat. "I'm tired now and want to go rest."

"Are you standing in the hallway again?"

"Yes. I want to go back and lie down."

"I can ask them to bring you a chair." Why wouldn't they have done that? Jackie had asked them to.

"No, it's okay."

"Can we get you a birthday gift? Your grandsons and I can send you a phone so you can talk to us from your room. We can also get you a digital picture frame with pictures of your family."

"No, thanks. I want to go now."

"Okay, the boys wanted me to tell you they love you. I love you, too."

"I love you, too. Bye."

And that was it. At least he could hear me this time. Other times when I phoned him and the staff brought him a cordless phone, he had difficulty holding it up to his ear and I'd spend the entire time saying, "Dad? Can you hear me? Are you there? Dad?" until I'd give up and hang up.

A few days later, Francine gave me another update. "I spoke with Jada today. The psych nurse practitioner will be in next Wednesday and will see your dad. Jada informed me that as of this Monday, he was refusing his medication. Of course they will continue to offer. I'm not sure how much effort they put into trying to persuade him. but his delusions likely don't allow much reasoning with him."

"Oh, only as of Monday?" I rolled my eyes. "I'm sure he's been spitting it out for a while."

"The nurses are pretty good at looking for that."

"They weren't when he was in the psychiatrist hospitals out here."

Francine changed topics. "Jada is going to ask the nurse practitioner to document Joseph's capacity to understand and sign a POA when she comes next week."

"I'm glad you're there to get info. Whenever I try to get a nurse on the phone, I'm transferred around and put on hold for a long time, only to be told that I need to talk to someone who either isn't there or is busy."

It turns out Francine wasn't getting much further than me, and that's with her actually being in Chicago. Perhaps because of short-staffing and high-turnover, there seems to be a universal problem with communication between medical professionals who care for patients with severe mental illnesses and the family members who try to remain involved in their treatment, because, in many cases, they're the twenty-four-hour caregivers.

Francine contacted me on July 25 with more information. "I've made several calls to the facility. Their responsiveness is variable. I finally spoke with Jada. I'd previously requested she ask the MD for a letter documenting capacity but that has not occurred. The psych nurse practitioner is coming next Wed AM. I plan to be there to meet her and hopefully get the document needed to move forward with POA."

"We need a letter that he's competent, so we can avoid going to court. And the sooner, the better." I was frustrated, but not with her, that it was taking so long. "Is Dad still refusing his medication?"

"I understand that while there are times when he refuses meds, he generally takes them."

"To be honest with you, I don't believe them. How can he be taking meds and not taking them?"

A week later, on July 31, Francine finally found some answers. She emailed me:

> I visited today and met with Joseph and staff
>
> 1) Joseph was discharged from therapy a couple weeks ago. He is now walking on his own and even takes the stairs to the therapy dept which I am told he visits periodically on his own to exercise
>
> 2). I believe the Wellbutrin twice daily was a transcription error. It was corrected mid-July. He is on 150 daily. He is on a small dose of Doxepin as a sleep aid, not in dose high enough to treat depression. The nurse practitioner was responsive and will write a letter re: Joseph's ability to understand POA document. She is to forward to me and I send to Melody.
>
> 3) Joseph invited me in and asked me to close the door so we could talk. He is very negative as you know. He indulged me in conversation about his circumstance and his choices. We had a good back and forth though no movement in his perception that he is a victim of his circumstances and things are hopeless. I do think that there was some progress in that he engaged. He told me I could return which I will do in a month. I also invited him to call me if he needed anything. "I don't talk on the phone," he told me. He looked good—clean shaven and wearing clean clothes.

I didn't know what she meant about him being a victim of his circumstance. She'd confirmed with me earlier that Dad continued to fear his enemies, which typically for him was the mafia. The meds were supposed to help with this paranoia. I couldn't do anything about it. Plus, he wasn't mentioning his paranoia to me.

An observation I've made over the years, is that oftentimes the best way to get improved care for a loved one—whether at a senior assisted living or other facility—is to frequently visit. If staff knows it's possible that a patient may have a visitor drop in at any time, they are more apt to make efforts to get the patient dressed or try harder to engage with them and follow their treatment more carefully.

I'm not saying that I believe staff in facilities try to neglect patients, but am simply noting human nature. If you have too many things to do at work, what task will you focus on first? The one the boss will be asking you about.

The answer I'd be seeking and we still didn't have an answer to yet, is whether or not my dad was deemed competent to sign the POAs. In the meantime, I kept worrying about where his pension was going or who was stealing it, and whether or not I'd be able to make medical decisions for him in the event of an emergency. The signed surrogate form only seemed to apply while he was there at his current facility, not if he was hospitalized.

Although Dad continued to refer to everyone there as "assholes," both to me over the phone and to Francine in person, she did her best during their visits to help him to reframe his negative outlook.

At the end of one of her visits, she noticed a birthday card which was signed by four staff members. She told him, "Not everyone is an asshole" and he agreed!

Now that I had an opportunity to redevelop a strained relationship with my dad, I wanted to help him in as many ways as I could. I sent Francine an email soliciting her help with this:

> A few concerns I have, in addition to medications:
>
> 1. I hope he can get his teeth checked and cleaned since he had complained his teeth hurt, especially when eating Sees chocolate I sent, which he used to enjoy.
>
> 2. I also wish he'd be willing to get glasses again. Then he could do crossword puzzles/ word searches/ other activity books / reading to keep himself busy and improve his mood. He used to like to read National Geographic magazines. I have a lot of them that I could send to him but I won't unless he has glasses and is

willing to read. He tends to throw things away now. I'm sure he's already thrown away the birthday cards my sister and I had sent him. I wonder if he still has the teddy bear.

3. He had mentioned to me on a phone call in January that he was worried he might be getting Alzheimer's, because he said his dad had it (which I was unaware of) and that he was forgetting some memories/things. If that's the case, I think there are medications to slow the progress of that so I'd like to know if Alzheimer's is a possibility. I do know that I took a genetic test that said I was predisposed to early onset Alzheimer's.

I wondered if there was any connection between signs of Alzheimer's and schizophrenia. Was there a way to tell when one ends and the other begins as far as impact on memories?

Alzheimer's is a form of dementia, which is what they listed on my grandma's death certificate as her cause of death, so it was likely part of our genetics. I pushed back my fears about getting Alzheimer's or, worse yet, late-onset schizophrenia. But nobody else in Dad's family had schizophrenia as far back as I was able to research. Besides, worrying about it wasn't going to change anything.

CHAPTER TWENTY-NINE

THE ENGAGEMENT

IN AUGUST, I traveled north to Sacramento with my good friend, octogenarian Jacquelyn (Jacki) Hanson, to sell books at the California State Fair. This was something we'd been together over the past few years. In one of the hangars that hosts the different California County displays, they have a section called California Authors. Months ahead of time, we had signed up for a few shifts. She'd grown up not far from there, so she made plans for us to stay with a friend of hers in the area.

I drove us up the 405 freeway to the 5 to the 99, surrounded by farmland and golden fields, while she related her fascinating life stories. Jacki was a spunky, petite retired public nurse who flew frequently with Liga International, Flying Doctors of Mercy to provide medical clinics in Mexico. She'd authored more than half a dozen works of historical fiction and had been a fixture at the fair for years—she had quite a few repeat customers.

In the morning, I dropped her off at the hanger, did the heavy lifting to bring everything in, then parked my car in the dirt exhibitor lot near the horse trailers. First thing I did after taking the shuttle back up is to go to the booth across from ours to buy a huge, sticky cinnamon bun for us to share—same as we did every year.

Although we did sell and sign books, we also seemed to be, as Jacki put it, part of the entertainment; she gave historical lessons while I provided emotional support and lent an ear to those who felt the desire to share after looking at my book, Losing Dad. Many individuals stopped to share their family's stories with me, and I was reminded how many people struggle. I'd see the pain behind their eyes. Sometimes they passed by me, speechless, because they were unable to share.

I signed each book with "Keep the Hope Alive." Now more than ever, these words hit home.

Later that afternoon, after buying a copy of my book, a woman looked at me with tears in her eyes, and said, "I'm so sorry for you and your family. Do you know where he is? Or if he's alive?"

"Mind if I share a spoiler with you?"

She nodded. "Please do."

"I found my dad." That was my first time saying those words in public.

"You did?" Joy lit up her face. "Are you writing another book?"

I hadn't considered it at that point. "Maybe."

"Can I give you a hug? What your family must've been through… I'm so glad you found him."

So, there I was, hugging a stranger like I'd often done before, but this time she provided comfort to me rather than me providing comfort to her. A moment of shared emotional connection.

I spent the day staring at the picture of my dad on the front cover and the framed family photos set up at my booth.

Human nature is to find others who can relate to our pain. Too often it seems hard to do when it comes to the burden, and unfortunately shame, of having a family member with a severe mental illness. It's not exactly the typical, "hey nice to meet you" conversation. With me, it was.

Rather than bask in the glow of finding him, the situation still felt a burden. I couldn't say, "hey, I found you," then put the facts away in a box up on a shelf. The worry I had for him was not as distant as it had once been. Now it was always in the background, like static. Sometimes I could tune it out, but occasionally, it would pop up again, like, "hi, remember me?" I knew his unhappiness and loneliness were things I couldn't cure with a pill or an occasional flight out there to visit. I couldn't solve his problems.

In August, Leo and I shopped for my anniversary gift. We had plans to celebrate our fourth anniversary with a weekend away up in Paso Robles at an inn on a vineyard, one of our favorite places. I couldn't wait.

"Do you know what you want?" Leo asked as we entered a jewelry store.

"Maybe an opal? I don't have any opal jewelry. Or maybe a sapphire?"

"What are you thinking? A ring?"

"Sure." He knew I loved jewelry for gifts—rings, necklaces, earrings.

We perused the display counters and I tried on a few here and there, but wasn't feeling moved by much. Leo led me over to the diamond displays where we found a beautiful setting of halo diamonds in white gold attached to an infinity band.

"A sapphire solitaire would be gorgeous in that," I said. "Don't you think?"

He smiled. "I do really like that one." He asked the associate to price it out.

But when the cost estimate came back for the sapphire, our jaws dropped.

"At that rate, I might as well buy a diamond." He turned to me and raised an eyebrow.

My stomach fluttered and I wrapped my arms around him and gave him a big kiss. "But you should know," I said, "that I'd like a better proposal than this."

He laughed. "I'm sure I can figure that out." Then he gave me a kiss.

I frantically phoned my insurance company to get the ring insured. Leo said we couldn't get engaged, because he wouldn't leave the house with it, until it was insured. I explained the dilemma to my agent who asked a manager to intervene to get it insured in record time.

On Friday, August 16, 2019 in Harmony Headlands Park, we stopped for our usual hike alongside the ocean. The parking lot was mostly empty as was the trail that day. I paused in front of trailhead sign and read about all the potential dangers that lie ahead. I pointed to the picture of a tick.

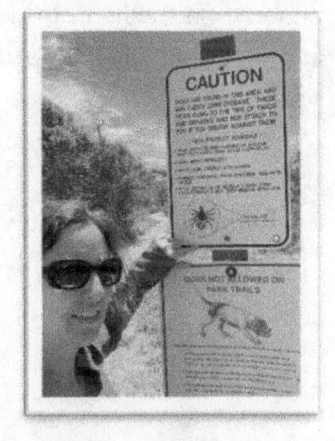

"I better not get any ticks." I shivered from the thought.

"You're not going to get a tick." Leo shook his head.

A light cool breeze brushed along my skin as we meandered along the path between hills and grasslands. Squirrels, lizards, and beetles darted in front of our feet.

I stopped to take pictures of the yellow California buttercups, golden poppies, lupine, and pink flowers bursting from round prickly bulbs, which Leo called wild artichokes.

He broke off a piece of anise. "Chew on this. It's the one that tastes like black licorice."

I did and pointed at a hawk circling overhead, more majestic than the turkey vultures nearby. The hawk squawked and flew higher and higher.

Leo and I rounded the bend. The grasslands and hills gave way to coastal scrub and bluffs. At the end of the trail, we sat atop a rocky outcrop. Waves crashed over the tidepools down below. Would this be the moment? I leaned my head against his chest and focused on the roar of the ocean and the sea lions on distance rocks jutting up from the sea.

Leo smacked his hand across my back. He stood up and grabbed my hands. "Come on, let's go back to the benches."

"What was on my back?" I jumped to my feet. "Was it a tick?"

"No." He led me away. "Just a small spider."

I shrieked. "Oh my God!" I hated spiders. Well, pretty much all bugs in fact. Surprisingly, I learned this from my dad. Hilda used to be the bug killer in our house, definitely not my dad.

Leo led me to a bench overlooking the ocean where he took out the ring and proposed. The diamond solitaire and halo of diamonds sparkled rainbows in the light. I threw my arms around him. Joy warmed my heart and we kissed. He wrapped his arms tighter around me and kissed the top of my head.

Back in the car, Leo turned to me and said, "By the way, it was a tick. A pretty big one."

I cringed. "No! I told you I didn't want ticks!" I examined my skin.

"Don't worry. I'll protect you from the nasty ticks."

At the inn, the employees celebrated our joy by bringing us, in addition to freshly baked chocolate chip cookies, a plate of chocolate-covered strawberries and two flutes of champagne.

After the joy settled in, my next thought was, I wanted Dad to meet my fiancé. I asked Fracine, "Do you think it would be possible for Dad to walk me down the aisle at my wedding?"

"Well, he is walking better," Francine said.

"Dad walked Jackie down the aisle at her wedding, so maybe he could do the same for me. When I got married the first time around, Dad wasn't around and Keith walked me down."

But this time could be different, I told myself. Dad could be included in our lives.

CHAPTER THIRTY

THE MISSING YEARS

FINALLY, IN AUGUST, Francine sent me and Melody the letter from the doctor that we'd been waiting for: the competency letter. This meant we could schedule the signing of the POA docs. I also received another document I'd been waiting for: Dad's admission records.

The sense of relief was short-lived when I read the competency doc:

> Joseph has been a patient of mine for the past 3 years. Throughout that time his mental status has varied, but it has been stable for the past 4 months. I did a decisional capacity evaluation on July 31, to evaluate his decisional capacity in regards to a POA. After I provided education, he was able to tell me the role that a POA plays in healthcare. He was also able to state that he would like his niece to fulfill that role, should it become necessary. She is currently serving as his surrogate decision maker. At the time I evaluated him, his thought process was goal oriented and he was alert and oriented x 4. He was not experiencing any audio or visual hallucinations, nor was he delusional.

Three years? That couldn't be right. Not to mention, clearly, I wasn't his niece. I scanned over the admission records. My eyes stopped at the top. Admission Date: October 2016.

It was, in fact, two months shy of three years. I sat in disbelief.

I had assumed maybe he'd only been there for a couple months. I vented to Jackie who was horrified. Keith said the system was obviously fucked up. I couldn't agree more.

Francine, Melody, and I got on a conference call to discuss the letter.

Francine asked, "Isn't Amanda his health surrogate?"

"Yes, it's supposed to be me," I said. "Shouldn't it specifically name me?

"Does he even have a niece?" Melody asked. "What about financial POA?"

"No," I said, "he doesn't have a niece, unless we count Hilda's niece whom he hasn't talked to in twenty years. He's an only child."

"My concern with how this letter is written," Melody said, "is that it appears as if he is confused or doesn't know that he doesn't have a niece. It is not an issue that she put in the letter who he wanted to name, just that he refers to her as his niece. Also, since the doctor chose to specifically mention health care, I don't want there to be any confusion regarding his ability to make financial decisions."

"Does that mean he's not mentally capable or that she's mixed up her information?" I asked. "Also, does it matter that it incorrectly states my dad has been her patient for three years, since the admission paperwork says he was admitted in October of 2016?"

"I think she either needs to re-do this letter or clarify it if we are going to rely on it."

"I don't understand how things that seem so simple can continually go so wrong," I said. "Even with the mental illness, I seriously doubt Dad has ever referred to me as his niece."

We sent the letter back to be fixed.

In the meantime, the realization hit me that Dad had been there in that facility by himself without a single visitor for two-and-a-half years until I found him. Incredible. How could no one have reached out to find his family? Is this common practice, to lock someone up in a jail or mental hospital, or other facility and never notify the next of kin? If so, it was a lousy policy.

But then that also meant that when I phoned the homeless shelter to try to locate Dad, that the manager there hadn't seen my dad in over two years, yet he remembered who he was well-enough to tell me he left in an ambulance? Does that mean he knew my dad well? If so, how long had Dad been at the shelter?

I kept backtracking time in my head, which only raised more questions.

His apartment lease—the one his parents prepaid a year on while they were still alive—expired on September 30, 2006. He would have been sixty-three, not yet old enough to claim social security at the time.

I didn't know where he went after that. I had tried to convince him to renew his lease but, because of his paranoia, he had refused. He asked my help in finding another apartment, but there was nothing he could afford with his income and without having the standard lease requirements and documents.

Later, on June 15, 2008, in a bizarre update, Dad showed me a dating profile that he'd posted online. He attempted to find a partner willing to preach on the streets with him. I couldn't take him seriously; as far as I knew he was still married to Hilda.

Then after one final call in 2009, he dropped off everyone's radar and disappeared.

Where was he from then until October of 2016?

It's strange to have a seven-year gap in history to where you can't explain where you've been or what you've been doing. I hated not having these answers.

I thought of when Hilda received the anonymous phone call in 2013 from the whispering stranger relaying the ominous warning that Dad was being taken advantage of.

Did Dad's old dating profile lead him to a scammer? I imagined my dad imprisoned in someone's basement while they stole all of his money. With his delusions and hallucinations, I imagined it wouldn't be hard for horrible people to manipulate or hurt him.

If it were true, how had Dad escaped? I knew his being imprisoned in someone's house sounded outlandish, like something out of a movie. But, as I learned long ago, anything was possible.

But was there any way to find out?

CHAPTER THIRTY-ONE

Keep the Hope Alive

Thank goodness for Francine. On September 25, 2019, the doctor sent a revised letter with me correctly listed as his daughter. I wondered if the doctor had reused a letter rather than typed up a new one? Not that it mattered at this point, because they'd redetermined Dad was medically competent enough to understand what he was about to sign.

And he did.

Melody met Francine there at the facility to notarize the signatures. Now it was official, as recognized by the state of Illinois.

"We need you to sign a few other docs because of the Patriot Act, including your ID and some other forms," Melody said. "Then I'll get you set up to receive monthly statements. We will now be able to take direction from you on your father's behalf for requests from the trust."

"No problem," I said. "I'm just so glad we've crossed this hurdle. How was he?"

"He looks very good and seemed to be in a good mood today. It's clear that he wants you to be the person making decisions for him. Francine will continue to visit with your father on a regular basis. He did agree that she could speak with the health care providers. We also discussed buying him some shoes and perhaps a winter jacket. He did tell us he is not allowed to leave without permission or with someone."

"If they let him leave, none of us would ever hear from him again." I sighed. I felt a weight lifted off my shoulders. Now, perhaps I could get some answers. "We do want to get him relocated to a better facility."

"Francine and I did discuss that. I think her first priority is talking to the medical staff and making sure that your father is being properly medicated. An issue we may run into is finding an appropriate facility for your father. It'll depend on his primary diagnosis. I'm sure Francine will discuss this with you more once she gets more information, which now she will be able to do."

Great. Another hurdle. I didn't stop to consider that not all senior living centers would accept patients with severe mental illness diseases. Yet another restriction was to find a place that accepted Medicaid payments.

"So, Dad could be stuck there, is that it?"

"No, I don't think so. Although the facility isn't the best, your dad does seem to be well taken care of and he seems to appreciate being there. When I asked him if there was anything he wanted or needed he said they gave him everything he needed there. We had to convince him to allow Francine to get him new shoes and a coat."

Oh, the "they're all a bunch of assholes" sentiment must not have been a thought Dad felt comfortable sharing with Melody. That and the constant turnover and inconsistent messaging from the staff regarding his medicine in particular.

"I'm going to get in touch with his pension company and I need to figure out which bank he was using. Did you say you were depositing money into an account for him?"

"Yes, monthly, until we stopped hearing from him."

"Which company?"

"Citibank."

"There's a branch ten minutes from me. I have a NAMIWalk this weekend and a lot going on at work, so I'll reach out to them as soon as I can and will keep you posted."

The annual NAMIWalk in Orange County was on Saturday, September 28, 2019 at Angel Stadium in Anaheim. My Walk Team, Kermitted to Kindness, raised money. Some students from our NAMI On Campus High

School Club joined my team, while others signed up to volunteer. This would be my first Walk since finding Dad.

I set up my books *Losing Dad* at a table to sell and autograph alongside old family photos featuring me and my dad. Ever since the publication of the book, I've donated a portion of the proceeds to NAMI OC, because I support their mission to raise awareness and offer education and support to families and individuals affected by mental illness.

Some people who had already read my book stopped by to say hi. I was thrilled to tell them I'd found my dad. I gave out so many hugs. If one family has a success, we all celebrate it. It's a beautiful community that helps you to know you are not alone in the struggle.

For some who bought the book, I asked their permission before offering a spoiler and told them the incredible news. For others, we agreed that they'd read the book first then check out my Instagram or Facebook pages to find the updates I'd posted.

One woman stopped and stared at the cover of my book then at the photos on the table. "Is that your dad? Are you Amanda?" After I nodded, she said, "I think I've met your dad."

"What? How?" I asked. "When?"

"We were searching on the streets for my son. I don't remember which city. But the man looked just like your father."

"He's been homeless throughout Chicago, Florida, Atlanta, and other cities. He believed he was a 'Prophet of God.' Was he preaching to you?"

"Yes, I believe so. Really nice guy."

I stared at her in disbelief. "That's incredible. Did you find your son?"

"Well…" She paused. "That's a long story. Eventually, yes. But he's not doing so well." Tears welled in her eyes and she touched the book cover. "I think it was your dad though."

"I'm so sorry." I recognized the all too familiar pain and suffering. "I hope the best for you, your son, and your family. Does your son still speak with you?"

She nodded. "But he won't get treatment."

I picked up my book and pointed to the cover. "The Foreword to my book was written by Dr. Xavier Amador. He explains the neurological condition of anosognosia, which is the inability to understand you're ill. He wrote about it in his book *I'm Not Sick, I Don't Need Help*."

"Never heard of it." She broke into a sad smile. "But that's a familiar phrase."

"I highly recommend his book. He teaches strategies on how to partner with a family member or loved one to get them treatment, without having to convince them that they're ill."

"How does that work?"

"It's counterintuitive to be honest with you. The good news is though, if you still have a relationship with your son, there's still hope."

She pursed her lips together and scrunched her face to hold back tears.

"Would you like a hug?" I asked.

She nodded and held out her arms. We met for an embrace, a moment of shared understanding. It's easy for people to say words of comfort, but far harder to get them to understand, unless they've walked in your shoes. Lived experience makes empathy possible. It brings comfort in the ways that a visit to a doctor can't always do.

She stood back and wiped her eyes. "Thank you. I'll get his book. And how much is yours? I'd like to get one, too."

"Twenty dollars for the paperback, but I'm sold out of the hardcovers." I handed her a copy. "Would you like me to autograph it?"

"Yes, please."

I signed, same as I always did, with the phrase "*Keep the Hope Alive!*"

After she paid and received the book, she stared into my eyes. "Thank you. I hope you find your father."

"I did. I found him in Chicago. After ten years, we finally found him."

"Really? That's incredible."

I pointed to my signature line "Your son is still talking to you. Anything is possible. Keep the hope alive."

"Thank you." She took a deep breath and departed with her head raised a little higher.

And this is why I wrote the book. And this is why I sell them in person—to have these conversations, to provide empathy, to inspire hope. Because without hope, what do we have left? Despair. If I can ease one person's suffering, even a little bit, when I sit at a table selling and signing books, then I feel my purpose has been fulfilled.

Everyone is on a different part of their journey, and no two journeys are the same.

CHAPTER THIRTY-TWO

The Shoes

In October, the weather chilled and the leaves were vibrant with color. Francine tried again to bring my dad shoes.

"I visited your dad this early afternoon," Francine told me. "He looked very good, just had a haircut. I brought him two pairs of shoes from REI but neither fit."

"Sounds about right." I laughed.

"Well, the good news is that he didn't protest that he didn't need them. I told him I'd been unsuccessful twice in bringing him shoes and I suggested we needed to shop together, so he can try on the shoes."

"To actually take him out?"

"Yes. And he agreed and told me, "I need a coat. I explained the—"

"Wait. He agreed?" How could he refuse to go out to museums or even dinner with me and my sons, but agree to leave to go shopping with Francine? I tried not to overthink it.

"Yes. He told me, 'You're doing too much for me.' I told him he deserved to have people help him and I hoped he would realize that. So, we have a date to shop and have lunch on October 24th. He told me barbecue would be fine but added, 'I like other things, too.'"

"He agreed to lunch, too? I don't know what magic you're performing if you can get him on an outing. What a huge accomplishment. When I talk to him on the phone, he never wants to speak for more than a few minutes. I don't think he likes standing up, even though sometimes I insist that the nurses get him a chair, but he soon says he's tired and asks to go back to lie down."

"He's doing better, it seems. I decided to wait to talk to the psych NP. I want to see how the 24th goes before we mention alternative meds. Perhaps some attention is the best medicine."

Maybe she was right. That was the magic—Dad finally had a regular visitor. Once you know what you're missing, it's harder to let go of it.

But could I move him out to a facility in California, so that he could have regular visits from family? Probably not. For one thing, it's hard enough to move a parent who is in a Medicaid facility from one county to another within the same state, much less from one state to another. The other issue is that no matter what, Dad always returned to his hometown, Chicago. He loved the Autumn colors and the change of seasons, possibly out of nostalgia. Ultimately, the decision was only Dad's to make.

When I asked, he adamantly insisted he stay in Chicago. So that's what had to happen.

I hoped Dad wouldn't cancel on Francine. I wouldn't be surprised if he did.

Leo and I had already begun planning our wedding and had chosen both a date and location: June 27, 2020 at a lovely regional park filled with hiking trails. Our first date had been a hike in 2015—I know how dangerous that looks from the outside but I didn't have the disapproving glare from my dad, who was missing, back then. I had shown up for the hike following the Boy Scout Motto of "Be Prepared" by wearing my scout green hiking pants, boots, a Camelback water pack complete with tube and straw, my hair in a ponytail pulled through my hat, sunglasses and sunblock on.

Leo, on the other hand, laced up his sneakers, held up his water bottle, and said, "You know we're just walking a couple miles there and back along the ridge, right?"

No, I hadn't known that, even though I had sent my GPS coordinates to a friend.

But here Leo and I were five years later, choosing colors for our wedding.

"Dad," I said to him during a phone call. "I'd like you to meet my fiancé, Leo."

"When?" Dad didn't ask much about him, because I'd already told him all the important details that I felt my father would want to know: criminal history, none; education, bachelor's in IT; employed, fulltime; credit score, great; kids, one son in between the ages of David and Justin.

"The wedding is in June. Unfortunately, he'll be out of vacation days this year, so we're thinking about flying out during my spring break in April."

"That's nice."

"Have you given any thought about if you could come out for my wedding?"

"I can't do that."

I had just found out that Keith and Abe had already committed to attending Abe's cousin's wedding out of the country, before Leo and I had gotten engaged. If Dad couldn't walk me down the aisle, and neither could Keith, I could ask Justin, but it felt a little weird to put him in that situation. At least we had eight months before our wedding to figure it out.

"Maybe you could record a speech or something," I said. "Francine could help you. That would be wonderful, but we don't have to discuss that now." I was dropping the hint for later.

But honestly, just having Dad meet Leo, and want to meet him, was more than I could have ever hoped for, especially because for so long, I had assumed Dad was dead.

I couldn't believe how lucky I was to have been given this second, third? fourth? chance to reconnect with Dad. This time, I felt confident I wouldn't lose him to the streets, again.

He was safe and secure in his facility.

Thank God. Or the universe. Or both.

CHAPTER THIRTY-THREE

GETTING NOWHERE

I FELT WE had already made so much progress with Dad's medical care, but I had to finish taking care of his finances before we could look into moving him to another facility.

After a long hold, I connected with a representative from Dad's pension company and explained the situation. "So, he's at a facility and I need to have his pension sent there to help pay for living expenses."

"I can't confirm whether or not your dad has a pension with us," the rep said.

"I already know he does. His wife gets the other half."

"Look, ma'am, I am unable to share any information with you unless you have our POA forms filled out."

"Why would I have to fill out your forms? I have legal documents from the state of Illinois. I believe you're required to accept these."

"No. This is company policy."

"What's the point in filling out and notarizing legal forms from the state if they aren't good enough for you? That doesn't make any sense."

"I can't say anything else other than that's the policy."

"Do you understand my dad is at a facility? I'm not asking for his money. Legally, because he's on Medicaid, any income needs to go to them.

Are you telling me that I have to get another notary to go and sign additional documents? I live across the country."

No matter what I said, they wouldn't budge. The illogic of the situation was mind blowing. What a stupid policy. State forms should supersede a private company's.

Unfortunately, Dad's former employer had been bought out by a British company and I wondered if that was part of the problem. I conceded defeat. Melody said she'd work on it.

Next up, I phoned Citibank.

"Where did your father open up his account?" the service agent asked.

"I don't know. I'm assuming a branch in Chicago. Why?"

"You're going to need to go in person to talk to them."

"In Chicago? Are you out of your mind? I'm in California."

"That's the branch that will handle this."

"Are you hearing what you're saying to me? Your bank has hundreds of branches."

The person couldn't fathom the problem, so I escalated to a manager and was told to talk to another department. That department transferred me to another special department.

The only thing that was consistent was that every person I spoke to gave me different directions.

On another day, I got lucky. I spoke to a person who knew the procedure. "Okay, here's what you can do. Mail a copy of the POA and two different IDs for yourself and a letter explaining the situation. It will go to the legal department and we can go from there."

I did so. I sent the copies, certified return receipt.

And I waited two weeks as instructed.

When I phoned back, an agent said, "We will only accept Citibank's POA form."

"Are you kidding me? No, that's untrue. You are an American company and this is a document recognized by the state of Illinois. I did what I was told to do. I sent everything to your legal department. I will not fill out your POA forms, too."

"Then we can't help you. That's the company policy. I can't give you any information."

I said a few choice words before hanging up.

Ready to yank out my hair, I visited a local branch instead. Maybe I'd have better luck speaking to an actual human being in person.

I brought the Illinois POA documents with me and queued in line to speak with a teller. That person referred me to one of their personal bankers, one who had their own cubicle with a desk and chairs and a potted plant. That individual had me wait to speak with the manager.

The amount of hours being wasted on something simple annoyed me. I understood the importance of protecting a person's financial accounts. I knew there was fraud and identity theft and scammers who stole people's money by coercing them to sign over their life savings.

But clearly, this was not one of those situations. I could give them the name of the doctor and facility if they wanted to confirm the validity of my claims. They could look up Laurie's legal license and speak with her. They could confirm that the notary was a real person. What was the basic issue, then?

"I'm sorry," the manager said, "we can't give you access to your dad's accounts."

"Even with these legal documents? What on earth is the point of filling out a financial POA if nobody will recognize that? I just can't accept that."

"Have you tried filling out the Citibank POA doc?"

I tried not to cry out of frustration. "Come on, I can't be the only person going through this. Think about it. It's a state approved document. I already sent it to your legal department."

He sighed. "Have a seat. Let me see what I can do."

I watched while he was given the runaround from his corporate office and bounced around to different people as well. The patience in his voice was wearing thin. If nothing else, it satisfied me to know I wasn't the only one getting jerked around by this nonsense.

Time ticked by. The branch employees locked the door and counted out their drawers.

The manager hung up the phone. "It looks like the person I need to speak with has left for the day. He handed me his business card. "I'll personally take care of it. I agree it's ridiculous. Can you stop by on Friday? We should have it all straightened out by the end of the week."

Right. Like I hadn't heard that before.

CHAPTER THIRTY-FOUR

The Outing

THURSDAY, OCTOBER 24, 2019

I was pleasantly surprised that Dad hadn't canceled his lunch outing with Francine. That afternoon, after returning Dad to the facility, Francine emailed me an update:

> I was delighted to find your father ready to go at 9:45 this AM. He practically jumped out of the bed! Fortunately, it was a beautiful day, and the leaves, still colorful. He was happy to be out and see the colors and the lake.

The first time in years Dad had been able to experience the reds, yellows, and oranges of the fall foliage, and Lake Michigan—two of his favorite things. I was thrilled Dad got to experience some of his fondest memories of the Midwest, even if I couldn't be there with him. The email continued:

> We drove to REI and found a pair of Merrell shoes that were identical to the ones he had. He was very pleased.

Shoes, like I remembered, had always been a very important thing to him. I was sure their importance only grew from the miles and miles he walked every day when he didn't have a place to sleep at night. Good shoes and socks made the difference between blisters and foot injuries. I was glad this priority of his hadn't changed.

> We then had lunch at a nearby restaurant. Joseph was very talkative. I don't believe that I brought up the subject of a move to another facility today but had previously. He brought up the subject during the lunch and indicated that he was receptive to considering another place to live. I told him I would investigate options. I wanted to make sure it would be an improvement. When I asked what he might want in another place he said "nothing." I jokingly told him that that would be easy to find!
>
> We talked about a lot of things, including his parents and where he has lived.

These were the memories I wished I had been there to hear. It seems every time I lost a family member—grandmother, grandfather, or anyone else, my biggest regret was not hearing more of their stories. Each a glimpse into the past provided a bridge between generations, and each time they passed away, I felt that bridge had crumpled.

What did he tell Francine? Did he tell her how his mom would make his soup and let him watch TV when he came home from school? Did he relate how he loved baseball?

Did he tell her about the piano?

After my parents divorced, my mom, my brother, and I ended up with a piano in the house. I didn't know why because it only seemed to gather dust. Vaguely, I knew Jackie had gotten lessons, but she didn't care to continue. Even if I wanted them, money had dried up after the divorce. So, the piano sat ignored, a place to put decorative kerosene lanterns.

When I was twelve, I opened up the piano bench and found not only my sister's beginner lessons, but also some older sheets of music by Beethoven. Why on earth that was there, I hadn't the slightest idea. My mom didn't play. Nobody did.

So, one summer, because I did love the sound of piano music, I set a goal for myself—learn how to play this wooden piece of furniture. I took pains going through every beginner's song over and over again until I could read the basic notes and understand which note corresponded to which white and black key.

After a while, I got tired of playing Three Blind Mice and other such silliness. I opened up the sheet music and turned the page. Fur Elise by Beethoven. The chaos on the page was intimidating. I meticulously labeled the notes lightly with a pencil. And I tried it, one measure at a time, going back to the beginning over and over. I remembered hearing the song somewhere, maybe on the classical radio station or on a movie, and I loved it.

Eventually I wanted to show my dad. One afternoon when he came to pick up me and Keith for the weekend, I pointed to the piano and said, "Dad, can I show you something?"

He nodded and sat down.

My fingers shook. I'd been working hard and wanted him to be proud of my efforts. When I finished the first page and a half—that's all I could play so far—I turned to my dad.

He smiled and nodded. "Very good."

Then in a dreamlike state he approached the piano. I stood so that he could sit on the bench. He silently studied the book for a few minutes. I didn't know why. He suspended his hands in the air and tapped at a key or two and pumped the pedals.

I stared in curiosity, but didn't say a word.

His hands landed on the keys and massaged each note into a beautiful melody. My jaw dropped. Since when did my dad know how to play the piano?

In awe, I listened while he finished out the song. I clapped for him, but he didn't say anything. He didn't acknowledge the incredulity of the situation for me, but he did return my hug. At that moment, I didn't care if he was proud of me; I was proud of him. That was my dad.

But he never played for me again. That was the first and the last time. I wished I had asked him about it at the time and the years afterward.

During later phone calls with my grandma, before her passing, she told me her only child—my dad—had shown a natural talent for classical music, but he refused to play. He preferred baseball, which he wasn't as good at.

I don't know if Francine got these kinds of stories from him, or if he forgot the memories or she didn't remember the details, because, after all, it wasn't her dad. Her intentions seemed to be based less on getting him to recall all of his past and more on motivating him to care about life, as I could tell in the rest of her email:

> One of my themes was that, while he was seventy-six, he had living to do and I hoped we could make his life better. I told him I was concerned that all he did was lay in bed. I encouraged him to go to exercise at least 3 times/wk. He listened without becoming irritable or defensive.
>
> He was very polite and grateful, to me and to all the people we encountered.
>
> As the visit continued, he evidenced some paranoia. He discussed the mob and his feeling that he had to be very careful as he had gotten into trouble with them. It is hard to gauge how distressing his delusions are. He seemed very matter of fact and not at all upset. He wanted assurance from me that our conversation would be private. I know you won't reference our conversation with him. He also told me that individuals at the facility spoke unkindly (my word) to him.
>
> Your dad also spoke of the Bible and the Bible's imperative to be content with what one had. I told him having a few more things (a couple more pairs of pants, a nicer winter coat) would still be good to have.
>
> I know this is a quite disjointed report but in sum, we had a good visit. I am hopeful that we can, in time, find a better setting. I am so pleased that your father is finding some small sense of possibility and some pleasure.

This was excellent! Francine had succeeded in getting Dad out for the day. It gave me hope that Dad could improve. Maybe the next time I flew out to visit him, he'd allow me to take him to lunch, or even a museum.

It's amazing how we can take the simplest things for granted. When a family member struggles with their mental health, any little victory can mean so much—be it getting out of bed, taking a shower, brushing teeth, and in this case—trying on a new pair of shoes in an actual store.

This was Dad's first time in over three years that he left the confines of the facility.

I stepped outside on my front porch. Wind brushed against my bare skin and shook the branches of my Sycamore tree. Leaves fluttered down to the green grass before a breeze swept them up and twirled them in a dance across the yard. Birds chirped and swooped in the distance. I imagined Dad experiencing all of this again—his love of nature, a love I, too, shared.

I delivered the good news with Keith and Jackie.

I didn't know what to expect from the future. But apparently, anything was possible.

CHAPTER THIRTY-FIVE

GAINING ACCESS

FRIDAY, OCTOBER 25, 2019

After work, I rushed through traffic to get to the Citibank branch before it closed. I hoped for the best but was prepared for the worst. I knew better than to get my hopes up. Why should anything logically go as it should? Life, for me at least, was never that simple.

But when I stepped foot inside, the manager spotted me, gave me a warm smile and waved me over.

"We got it all taken care of," he said. "Have a seat."

I wanted to cry tears of relief and joy. "Thank you so much. I really appreciate your help. I just want this all to be done."

"Do you have some time right now? We can get you set up on the account, get you an ATM card and set up the pin, and get you going with online access. But it will take a while."

"Wow. Of course." As if I'd leave and risk losing the possible progress being dangled in front of me.

It did take a while, over an hour.

"This is only a temporary card." He handed me a blue debit card. "You'll get another one in the mail. I've changed the address as well. You shouldn't have any issues going forward. Is there anything else I can do for you?"

"How do I sign for him?"

"Sign your name, then write the words 'POA for', then sign his name."

"Can you print out his bank statements for me?"

"I'm not here tomorrow, but if you want to come back on Monday I can. They've already locked up for the night." He tapped away at a computer. "To be honest with you, other than that pension you mentioned, there hasn't been a single transaction in the last two years. Online, you should be able to go back seven years, so that would bring you back to 2012."

2012. That meant I could potentially track Dad through his purchases.

"Never mind then," I said. "I'll go home and check it out online."

"Call me or come by if you have any issues at all."

While I drove home, I realized that because of my exhaustion, I hadn't even asked for the bank balance. How stupid of me. Until I could sit down at my computer, I wouldn't know if he had ten thousand dollars in there, with three years of pension payments accumulating.

His pension. I thought of the pain in ass I was getting from his company. Screw you. I knew he had a pension.

At my computer, I registered for online access to Dad's account. Set up the security questions. Yada yada. I looked at the date: Friday, October 25. This had taken an entire month from the date Dad had signed the POAs to get straightened out. Way too long, but at least the stress was finally over with.

I verified my email address.

At last, the website allowed me to log in.

And then I saw his bank balance.

Shit.

PART THREE

COMPLICATIONS (2020-2021)

CHAPTER THIRTY-SIX

Forensic Accounting

I BLINKED AND stared at the numbers on the screen: $116,170. $116,170!

What the actual fuck.

We were screwed.

It was too late Central Time to phone Melody, so I wouldn't be able to reach her until Monday. That meant I wasn't going to sleep well.

Now I know under normal circumstances, finding a hundred grand tucked away in a bank account would seem like a miraculous gift from the heavens. But these weren't normal circumstances. I immediately understood the serious implications of this.

I agreed to act as his POA. I had a legal obligation to handle his finances.

And this was *clearly* well over the two-thousand-dollar asset limit for Medicaid coverage. Medicaid paid for the facility. If I didn't do something soon, this could be considered Medicaid fraud punishable by prison and or huge penalties and fines. Granted Dad didn't commit fraud on purpose—he didn't even remember he had a bank account.

But the difference was that now that I knew about the money, I had to deal with it.

Dad's medical coverage could get dropped. Would they dump him back on the streets if he didn't have insurance coverage?

How did this happen?

I downloaded all of Dad's bank statements for as far back as I could to try to piece together his life. October 2012 was the oldest one I could access.

He had income from social security, his small pension and a monthly deposit from the trust company.

Then again, some people who live on the streets with untreated severe mental illnesses have a lot of money, like the millionaire whose family desperately kept trying to get her into housing with the help of the Orange County Sheriff's Missing Persons Department. No matter how many times they tracked the woman down and tried to get her help, without treatment for the SMI, she returned to a life of transient homelessness.

It was perplexing to hear about the hoarders or the transient individuals who, after their death, were found to be wealthy. SMI does not discriminate. No matter how much money a person has, SMIs are, at least to date, incurable. But they are treatable. Sometimes, but not always.

What havoc had the SMI done on Dad during his missing years? I searched for clues on his bank statements.

As far as bills... No automatic bill pays.

But there were cash withdrawals. A lot of them.

The number of cash withdrawals, many in odd amounts, made no sense to me.

There were precise amounts withdrawn from a teller like $469.64 and $435.64. Then there were amounts like $700 taken out from tellers or the ATM every few days. How was he burning through so much cash?

Had someone indeed been taking advantage of him? Or was he living out of hotels?

Besides social security and his pension checks—which should have been six times as much had he not taken his pension so early because of his SMI—there were also additional transfers from the trust throughout some months, seemingly at random. And there were a couple outlier deposits, like $312.36 cash deposited through a bank teller. Who deposits $312.36 in cash?

Where was he during that time? In 2015, the automatic monthly transfers from the trust increased slightly, but all of the other random transfers from them stopped. I was surprised he hadn't completely drained the trust already at that point.

It disturbed me whenever I heard on the news an elderly person was being held hostage while someone else, often someone who had gained their trust, stole their life savings. Maybe this had been the case with Dad.

Maybe this discrepancy in deposit activity was an indication that one or more individuals had siphoned money from Dad. These large transfers could provide evidence to back up that claim, but because everything came out in cash, there was no paper trail to follow. Because so many years had passed, there wouldn't be any video evidence either.

Except for a few transactions in Chicago, most statements did not report where his withdrawals were occurring, so, unfortunately, I couldn't track his location as I had hoped.

By mid-2015, the ATM and teller withdrawals sometimes jumped up to $1100 at a time and deposits—one for $12.36, for example—were erratic.

That's when another pattern jumped out at me: Dad had consistently maintained a balance that ended with zero cents. In fact, almost every transaction left his account rounded to the nearest hundred, like $1400.00. Nothing but four zeros at the end. No cents. Unusual. I didn't know anyone else who obsessed over those kinds of details.

Because he never used credit cards—he hadn't done so when I was a kid, either—and he hadn't done any Point-of-Service purchases at any stores or restaurants, he must have paid for all housing and food and transportation through cash.

I remembered when I traveled through Chicago and New York City with him, he had bought me a one-way ticket to NYC by paying cash at the reservation counter. That landed us being flagged for extra security pat downs in the security checkpoint.

If he'd been paying everything in cash, how many suspicions would that have raised? Would he have been on anyone's radar? Was he robbed? Mugged multiple times?

I imagined carrying thousands of dollars on your person wasn't the safest idea. But for someone as paranoid as he was, who believed the Mob and the FBI were after him, perhaps it made sense to him. It would have been ironic if the FBI were tracking him because of all of his large cash transactions.

I continued to scour through his statements.

On June 1, 2015, city data showed up. All withdrawals at that point originated out of Florida, the other place I knew he'd been frequently in the past. There were various cities including Miami, Coral Gables, Ft. Lauderdale, Surfside. I couldn't feel too bad for him if he was enjoying these locations, but was he alone? He was burning through a lot of cash.

In September 2015, withdrawals continued, but the location information disappeared.

Maybe he had gone back to Chicago in preparation for winter? But why, if he had the money and choice, would he stay in Florida for the summer, and return to Chicago for the freezing winter? It was illogical.

No city information existed on the rest of the numerous withdrawals. Each transaction from September 2015 through June 2016 happened in mystery locations.

But in July 2016, the city data on one single transaction confirmed he was in Chicago. In August 2016, a few transactions showed he, or at least his ATM card, was in Wisconsin. Who did he know in Wisconsin? In September, according to one random record, he or his ATM card was back in Chicago.

Then, on September 26, 2016, after two withdrawals of $803.50 and $796.50 on Diversey Parkway in Chicago—to even out the bank balance with four zeros at the end for the tens, ones, and cents—the transactions abruptly stopped.

Not a single withdrawal occurred after that date.

Thus, his account accumulated a balance at that point.

Perhaps that's when he ended up in the homeless shelter in Chicago, the one whose manager I had spoken to when trying to track Dad down. If he'd been living out of a shelter any earlier than that, there would have been no explanation for the cash spending happening every few days. Only a hotel could require that amount of expenditures.

Dad had been admitted to the nursing home facility on October 19, 2016.

And that was the last day he physically left the facility. I wondered if he felt like he was forced to stay inside like a prisoner. But if they had outings when they did activities, I'm sure Dad would have never agreed to go, instead sinking inward more, refusing to participate in the world outside him.

One final social security check was deposited in May 2017. Perhaps that's when his facility got his social security checks sent directly to them, seven months after he was admitted there as a patient, and eventually became a resident.

What was his first night like there? Was he scared? What kind of roommates did he have? Did he know where he was? That must've been a harsh transition to go from traveling through Florida and Chicago to ending up locked up there.

What changed? What happened after September 26, 2016? My mind came up with a million possibilities. Had someone attacked him the next day? Did he have another heart attack?

Since he'd recently told me he didn't even believe he had a bank account, I wondered how could someone who'd been taking out hundreds of dollars every few days magically forget he had one? Something major had to have happened to him. And because it wasn't in his current medical records and nobody who worked at the facility now was there when he was admitted, I'd never get those questions answered.

Sometimes, all you can do is let it go. Let things be. Contrary to what I'd learned, there wasn't always an answer for everything. Some things didn't make sense and I couldn't will the answers out of thin air. I could do the best I could with the information I had, but had to be okay with not knowing and not understanding everything else.

I looked through the rest of the bank statements. The automatic monthly transfers from the trust company had ended in May of 2018, which made sense considering they got in touch with me a month and a half after that. That had been the moment that had led to this moment.

In June 2018, Dad's account went dormant. The only reason the account had stayed open and didn't attract attention from the bank were the automatic monthly pension deposits.

Otherwise, his account could have been closed for inactivity and the money transferred to the Illinois State Controller. I knew. It'd happened to me before in California. I had an old credit union account I had forgotten about from college. I had to fill out the claim form to get my five dollars back.

It happened frequently enough that people didn't realize they had unclaimed money—perhaps a partial refund from a utility company after moving, or an insurance company refund after a policy was canceled, or any number of other scenarios. Now at least it was easy to check each state's online searchable database for unclaimed property through their official government websites. Type in the name and see what pops up. Maybe a few dollars here, a few dollars there.

What would have been the procedure if this had happened to Dad's account, which contained over a hundred thousand dollars? Would it have ended up in the court system? Would local authorities have gone searching for him, or tried to locate his next of kin? Would anyone had made a connection between that and the missing persons report? Or, would it have become just another searchable item, his name and account just another entry in their vast database?

Even though I couldn't precisely figure out where Dad had been from 2009 through 2016, I felt a sense of comfort in finding out what I had discovered so far. Being able to loosely track Dad financially over that limited time period, was like being a distant viewer of his life's activities. Rather than view vacation pictures posted to social media, I got to see his financial footprints.

Because I didn't get the normalcy of modern day living, of sending text messages, video chats, and reading his online updates in my social media feeds, this was the closest thing I had to a relationship with my dad during his years of absence.

CHAPTER THIRTY-SEVEN

SIGNS OF LOVE

By the time I woke up in the morning, ready to deal with the new financial crisis, another thought intruded my brain space: What if Dad hadn't been living on the streets during those years, at least from 2012-2016? Maybe he had been traveling on his free will, staying in lovely seaside hotels every night, not sleeping on park benches or sidewalks or shelters. Maybe it wasn't like before, like it had been before his parents died, before he cursed his mom on her deathbed. Back then, he very much slept on the streets.

On the one hand, it would be wonderful to know he hadn't suffered during that time.

On the other hand, if that were true, did that mean he didn't love his family? Had he purposely abandoned all of us? Did he care? Had he no longer loved his daughters and son, or wanted to get to know his grandchildren, to spend holidays with Justin and David?

Or, had the mental illness stripped his emotions and ability to remember he had family? Had the SMI damaged or destroyed Dad's ability to connect emotionally, with anyone at all? Was he relegated to merely transport through life rather than to truly live it?

It was hard not to take personally. I had to remind myself that mental illness doesn't care about you or them or anyone. This was not my dad. I firmly believed that. This was the SMI.

The Dad I remembered was the one who slipped me forty dollars when I was pregnant and needed money, but was too proud to ask. He did it when no one was looking. And he'd done it more than once.

My Dad was the one who, when my sister was in college and said "everything's fine," even though it wasn't, would casually open up her kitchen cabinets. Jackie didn't have anything other than a couple cans of soup and a box of mac n' cheese in her apartment, so he took her shopping. He loaded up her refrigerator and freezer, and filled her shelves. She didn't ask him for it. He just did it. And he didn't announce it to the rest of us.

Knowing when to help and when to standby was a fine line. Both were equally important. For the most part, even though no one's perfect, he did a pretty good job with the balance.

I promised I would be the same parent to my sons. If I ever saw them in need as adults, I'd step in and help them, quietly, without fanfare, because that's what I'd learned from my dad. That was the kind of dad he was. And that's the kind of mom I wanted to be.

That was the dad I knew and remembered and loved.

But I had to love this dad, too, the one who stayed in touch in his own strange ways via phone and letter and email. The one who sent me dozens of YouTube videos in a day then nothing for months. The dad who invited me to join him in adventuring across the streets of Chicago and New York City back in 2004, who showed me the sensitive fern and waited for my reaction. The dad who couldn't wait to show me fireworks off Navy Pier and took me to the Build-a-Bear store.

I realized that all those years, even though he was ill, Dad wasn't entirely disconnected emotionally. In his own way, he had loved me, just not in the way he'd been capable of before.

When a loved one develops Alzheimer's or dementia or a severe mental illness, the experience can feel similar. It's a pain in the ass and a thankless job to take care of the difficult person in front of you.

So, why do it? Why bother with all of the stress and headache?

Because you are thanking the person they once were. You are giving back the love they gave, which you were lucky enough to receive.

CHAPTER THIRTY-EIGHT

In Limbo

Over the weekend, the more I thought about it and reexamined the bank statements, the angrier I became. I hadn't realized the trust company's transfers were continuous up until May 2018. Didn't they have a fiscal responsibility to ensure he was housed and to safeguard his money? If they could do skip tracing and hire a traveling nurse, couldn't they have somehow investigated whether or not someone had been taking advantage of him? I'm sure my grandparents would have been furious. I ruminated on what may have happened to Dad during all of the gaps of time.

If we wanted to get Dad moved to another facility, we needed this resolved. I couldn't lie on his resident application under the financial section. It could endanger his current placement as well.

As soon as I awoke Monday morning, I phoned the trust company.

"How did this happen?" I asked Melody as I related the details from the bank statements. "Why were you sending him money every month without hearing from him? Didn't you all make him contact you? See if he needed anything? Check on him? This much money shouldn't have accumulated in his accounts."

"I'm sure it was his social security and pension, too," Melody said.

"Not this much!"

"Let me talk to some people here and get back to you."

But I shouldn't have gotten mad at her. My irritation and anger were misplaced. But it wasn't not like I could confront his SMI and beat the shit out of it. After so many times of sitting and taking it, it was hard not to feel like a punching bag with the repercussions of his serious mental illness constantly pummeling me from every direction—emotional, financial, medical, legal.

At times, despite my best intentions, I became enraged and exasperated with the world, but that was a part of what made us human—emotions.

When a person experiences the "negative" symptoms of schizophrenia, not the fear or anxiety, but the emotional flatness, it seems like the disease strips a part of the person's humanity, their ability to feel and to express those feelings in an appropriate way. So, family and loved ones are stuck experiencing frustration by their loved one's lack of emotions. It's painful to have to mourn the loss of reciprocal emotions. It's okay to be angry. Anger comes from hurt and pain. What's not okay is to take it out on others.

No matter what though, it was important to recognize that Dad wasn't deliberately causing me pain; it was his SMI. And mental illness is a brain disease, a problem with imbalanced chemicals in the brain. The brain is an organ as important as your heart and lungs. SMI is also a physical illness. Sometimes external factors and trauma trigger it; other times, it's hereditary. But stress can also trigger heart attacks and worsen the body's immune response to cancer among a bunch of other health ailments.

Mental illness is not a character flaw and it is not a choice. Who would choose it? And if it were you, how would you want to be treated? Would you want to be blamed for having cancer or diabetes or heart disease or mental illness? Highly unlikely.

So many thoughts swirled through my mind. Would we have to move Dad over to private pay, which was over ten thousand dollars a month (the current rate for his crappy housing)? That would be more than $120,000 in a year, or almost a million dollars for eight years. There was no way there was enough money in the trust to cover that. If the facility or Medicare or Medicaid found out, would he end up on the streets, again?

I told Keith and Jackie in a conference call.

"You know I'm not good at numbers," Jackie said. "But how could it possibly cost that much money for him to share a tiny room in that rundown facility? What's going to happen to Dad?"

"We can't afford to cover that cost," Keith said. "There's no way. I mean, I still can't mentally process how this could have happened in the first place."

"Me neither," I said. "Any suggestions?"

"I don't know," Jackie said. "But we can't let him lose his housing. He needs medical care."

"Well, obviously," Keith said. "I guess we'll just have to wait and see what the trust company says."

The next day, after Melody consulted with Candace, they advised me to hire a specialized attorney, one with extensive experience in the realm of Medicare and Medicaid. They gave me the phone number of a firm. The attorneys weren't cheap, but that didn't matter anymore. They could take all that money in Dad's account for all I cared. I just needed to know he wouldn't end up back on the streets.

Forget everything else. This was now on the top of my priority list.

Before I could pay the retainer fee to the law firm, I had to fill out their paperwork and await the attorney's direction. I discovered it was possible we might have to enroll Dad into the new facility under a private pay arrangement with the understanding that he was going to removed then re-enrolled in Medicaid as soon as we sorted everything out. But there were other possibilities they were looking at, so it was hard to know yet which way it would go.

Nothing moved as quickly as I had hoped. I spoke with the attorney's assistant, a Medicaid Consultant, Jill, several times as I tried to gather all of the documents that they needed for them to even begin to work on the case, including a copy of his social security statement and his Medicare ID.

Unless you've gone through this yourself for an elderly parent or a loved one with a SMI, it's hard to imagine how difficult it is to get documents, like multiple forms of ID, for someone else when that adult is unwilling or, as in our case, unable to get you what you need.

Much like with the financial organizations, it feels like nobody trusts you, not the social security department or Medicare or Medicaid or any other government agency. It feels like everyone assumes you're a thief trying to hack into accounts and steal money. Again, I know that's a very real issue. But, it's an incredible challenge to convince others that your intentions are pure and you're only trying to provide needed care for your loved one.

Everything takes forever. Endless patience and lots of time, both of which I was becoming increasingly short of. I had lesson plans to create, papers to grade, my own children to care for, and, now, a wedding to plan.

CHAPTER THIRTY-NINE

NORMALCY

ON SATURDAY, NOVEMBER 9, 2019, something happened that hadn't happened in over ten years: Dad phoned *me* and left me a voicemail. Voicemails—the things we take for granted and sometimes even delete before listening to the entire message.

I couldn't believe it. Dad had phoned me.

I pressed play.

"Okay, this is Dad," he said. "Just wanted to chat a bit. What was your fiancé's name? What does he enjoy doing? What do you enjoy doing? What does Justin like? What David likes? See, he likes art. He could do that as a teacher and then do freelance… Anyways, you're occupied now, so I'll hang up."

Everything about this message struck me as incredible—he remembered the names of both grandsons, he remembered I had a fiancé, and he even remembered David's interest in art.

Beyond that, there was another layer of unbelievable reality to his message. He was considering a potential job for David—this was a normal grandparent thing to do. My Dad was anything other than an average grandparent.

Plus, he brought up teaching. I hadn't realized, until my grandpa passed away, that I was a third-generation teacher. The year I was born, my dad's father retired from his career as a high school science teacher. His wife, my grandma, had been an elementary school substitute teacher.

My dad, before his career in IT, had taught high school math for a couple years, but I heard he was verifiably horrible at it. Back when Jackie needed help in Calculus, anytime she asked him for help, she ended up leaving the room screaming and crying. She said his intelligent brain was so up in the clouds that he seemed to overcomplicate everything. She couldn't get him to break things down in simple enough terms that she, someone who had no interest in math, could understand.

Later, she met a friend in college who said she had traveled to Israel and met another American from Southern California. The two girls got to talking about high school, with the new one relating a story about the worst math teacher she had ever had. After comparing details, Jackie later found out that this other girl had been referring to our dad. Wow. To be famous, and not in a good way, in another country.

Fortunately, my dad found his calling as a systems programmer and software analyst who worked on Mainframe computers for seventeen years in Pasadena. It was a much better fit for him.

And, I came to teaching as a second career. Initially, I graduated with a degree in business, worked in finance, but became disillusioned with the industry and decided to try my hand at teaching after several friends suggested it—I used to help them in school and apparently was better than my dad at patiently explaining how to do things.

So, three generations—science teacher, math teacher, and English teacher—and Dad was suggesting David consider taking up the noble profession. It felt surreal to see this part of Dad, the part that my entire family lost out on, but that was still, even if only a little sliver, there.

I didn't know if Francine had arranged a switch in Dad's medication, or if he was actually taking it, or if, like she suggested, some regular attention was currently the best medicine.

It didn't matter. Knowing how fleeting the present behavior could be, I treasured every minute of it, every time he said his grandson's name, and every time he expressed his love.

I returned Dad's call and had a relatively normal conversation, albeit short because he got tired of standing and wanted to go back to bed. This despite me asking them to bring him a chair. Still, we both ended the call with an "I love you."

I couldn't wait to tell Francine, but I got distracted with work. I had to spend hours scoring essays before grades were due. Finally, I sent Francine an email on November 13:

> Good news! Within the last week, my dad phoned me twice, including once when he left me a voicemail (this is the first time he's called in over ten years). He has discovered that he can go to the front office and ask them to call my number for him. He is asking questions about his grandkids and starting to discuss his lack of connection to his own family when he was a child. He's also indicated he wants to meet my fiancé soon.
>
> Whatever medication they have him on has made a tremendous difference. Thank you for all your hard work, Francine.

She responded: "I am so very happy to hear. I am not aware of any med changes, but he is seeing possibilities."

And yes, perhaps he was finally seeing the possibilities.

Dad phoned me again on Sunday, November 17. Our conversation was very short.

"I want to go lie down," he said.

"Well, I don't blame you if you're having to stand in the hallway to talk on the phone, or use the cordless phone that's so hard to hear you on. Why don't we get you a simple flip phone?"

"No, absolutely not."

"But you can have our phone numbers pre-programmed and call us whenever you want. That way you could be more comfortable."

"I don't want to mess with any technology."

I remembered his paranoia about the FBI and Mob and the five billion emails he used to send me from a thousand different email aliases because he thought people were tracking him. Perhaps it was best not to give him Internet access or technology that would increase his suspicions.

"Well, if you don't want a phone, is there anything else I can get you?"

"Could you get me some hard candies?"

"Like Werther's caramel, or butterscotch, or what?"

"That would be nice."

"Absolutely. I'll mail tomorrow." That was the first time he specifically asked me for anything at all. I wanted him to know he could depend on his family, that he could trust us. So, I bought them and mailed them out that same day.

With Thanksgiving coming up, knowing Dad would be without family—now that he knew we existed again—I worried this would exacerbate his depression.

Jackie, Keith, and I agreed to send a couple of boxes of See's Candy again—soft centers only this time now that I knew his teeth were bothering him. We send one for him and one box for the staff to share. Best to keep on their good side until we could find another home for him. Before submitting the order, I added a few of the butterscotch lollipops, too.

On November 21, I missed another call from Dad, but he left me another voicemail.

"Hi Amanda," he said. "This is Dad. I got the candy. Thank you very much." He gave a partial chuckle. "It's all gone now. Okay that's all I wanted to say, is thank you. Bye. Love you."

He got it, he loved it, and he loved me. And he was able to articulate all of that. And what's more impressive is that was the first time in a long time I had detected any hint of laughter from him.

My how far we'd come. I held onto hope that we could go even farther with his disease management and restore him to his former self, at least part of his old self.

CHAPTER FORTY

NEW PROSPECTS

In December 2019, Francine continued to talk in earnest to Dad about his options, a couple facilities she felt were a step up from his current one. She updated me on their visit.

Dad greeted her with "I hate this Goddamn place. But I don't want to move."

"Nobody is going to force a move," she told him. "I checked out a couple places and think one in particular is a definite improvement. Do you want to go see it in January? We can go to lunch afterward.

He agreed then added, "These clothes don't belong to me."

This was a recurring problem. Whenever we bought him clothing, even if we labeled the tags with his name, they disappeared after getting washed. He instead ended up with the same raggedy clothes that others had worn. I knew they had a lot of patients to keep track of, but didn't see why it was impossible to get his things back to him.

I've since noticed the same issues in other senior nursing homes with other family members, including most recently, my mom. If the family didn't take home their loved ones' clothes to wash, there was no guarantee they'd get back the clothing they bought. Any clothes seemed to become collective clothes and would disappear from their closets. This was especially true in the larger facilities. It was frustrating.

"We can buy you a pair of sweatpants and a zip-up sweatshirt," Francine told him, "Until we find you a coat you like, because you don't have any long sleeve shirts or socks."

He nodded.

"I'll bring you socks." Before leaving, she told him, "I want to assure you that I'm keeping Amanda informed. No move would be made without her input and approval."

"Good."

While Francine made appointments to tour the new facilities, I filled out paperwork on the backend in the evenings after work. But often I didn't understand how to answer some of the questions.

During lunch at work, I closed my classroom door, sat down at my desk, and called Francine.

"What level of care would you say my dad needs?" I asked. "Assisted living, memory care, or nursing home?"

"I don't believe that your father can live in Assisted Living. The only A.L. that accepts Medicaid in IL is called Supportive Living. They cannot take people with a primary mental illness diagnosis."

I wrote that in my notepad. "Seems to be the norm. By the way, I discovered it was more than his clothing going missing. With him sharing a bathroom with three other people, even his special toothpaste, the Sensodyne we bought him, went missing."

"That's unfortunate. He shares a bathroom with at least three other people. I don't know why these places can't manage to keep things straight. But if you have the receipts, we can ask them to reimburse you for any missing items. I didn't see his pillow there the last time either."

"Dad seems resigned to the fact that nothing he owns is guaranteed to be there in the morning. It's not okay."

"Well, there does seem to be more positive news. Your dad is calling me which makes me think he trusts me and sees me as an advocate. That's a good thing."

"And he phones me every couple of weeks. So much has happened this year and I thank you for everything."

"It's a lot to deal with. Let's get some of your concerns addressed ahead of time with the new place."

I hoped he could even get in a new place. I glanced up at the clock—only twenty minutes remained of my thirty-minute lunch break. My stomach growled but I also had to use the restroom. I took a bite of my peanut butter and jelly sandwich—David and I had made our lunches together the night before—and called Dad. Fortunately, I was able to get him on the phone right away.

After consulting with him, he and I came up with a list of questions he wanted me to ask the staff at the potential new facilities: Namely, would his shampoo, toothpaste, clothing, and personal items be kept private, or would they go missing?

Dad valued quiet time in his room and wanted to know if he'd be forced to room with someone who played the TV or radio or was noisy. Of course, we'd prefer he had a private room, but knew that was unlikely.

He also expressed concern regarding the quality of the food, and if he'd have multiple options per meal or be stuck with the same thing. Apparently at his current facility, his choices were not honored.

I came up with additional questions, which I didn't discuss with him, most for obvious reasons, namely that, thanks to the anosognosia, he still didn't believe he had a mental illness. I doubted Dad even believed they existed. So, I added information and questions to the list.

I told them that he didn't believe he had any psychiatric disorder, so I wanted to know how would the new facility be able to manage his medication, both his heart medicine and psychiatric medicine, under these circumstances. Because he'd complained about tooth pain in the past, I asked if he'd have good dental care there. Was that even covered under Medicare? I needed to understand how to get him medical, dental, and vision insurance coverage, supplemental Medicare plans, since he could end up be off Medicaid very shortly.

Concerned about the high turnover we'd experienced, I asked about that and if Francine and I would have access to social workers, psychiatrists, and psychologists to answer our questions. He needed access to the outdoors, free from cigarette smoke. I wanted him to be at a place that gave him opportunities for field trips and activities. I also asked if he'd be able to work on a regular basis with someone in the rehab department exercising so he'd be able to stand more than five minutes on a phone call with me without getting tired and needing to lie down again.

The school bell rang. Lunch was over. I realized I'd have to wait at least an hour before using the restroom, but at least I'd been able to send the email. One thing off the checklist.

I wiped my mouth, brushed the crumbs off my desk, and went to open my classroom door. I plastered a smile on my face and welcomed in the grumpy sixteen and seventeen-year-olds.

Fortunately, I got almost all those questions quickly answered by speaking to the admissions department at the facility. They only needed me to get his social security award letter and a referral letter sent from his current facility to get him moved. This, to me, was the best news ever. I requested a window bed—if Dad wanted one—and only one roommate, rather than three to four in a room.

The new staff assured me that they'd label all of his things when he got there as well as any new items purchases. He could lock his cabinet and dresser but they felt it would be unnecessary. Also, each room had its own restroom, so he'd only be sharing with any roommates. He'd be matched with other residents who preferred quiet time as well. Their menu included a variety of options, including daily specials and standard choices such as cheeseburgers, grilled cheese, and Indian dishes because they had a large Indian and Pakistani population. They would also work with the dietitian for his heart healthy meal plans.

And, in regards to my additional questions they told me that they had stable staffing, a psych nurse on staff every day and three psychiatrists that came by to check on patients. They'd relate all my concerns to the staff and the social workers, which were there every day. One Friday a month they brought in a dentist to do cleanings. If he needed any dental work, they'd take care of the transportation to get him to another location for the procedure.

As far as getting him outside, they had an outdoor patio accessible during good weather, smokers only had limited time to smoke out there, but even if they were out there, the patio was large enough for him to avoid that area. They also took up to fifteen patients at a time on a bus on outings.

If he wanted something from a restaurant, it could be brought back for him as well.

Patient rooms were upstairs and downstairs they had an activity room, dining room, and lobby. He could also go out on passes any time with Francine or family.

I was glad to find out that patients had phones at each bed, but the recommendation was that we get him a basic phone with prepaid minutes or when he was back on Medicaid possibly get him a lifeline phone, which was a free cell phone like my mom had.

I appreciated the suggestion, but had a feeling that Dad still wouldn't agree to the phone.

Because I understood that this might be the only time that I'd be able to move Dad to a new facility, I wanted more specific information to make sure I was choosing the best place possible. Francine had mentioned another place, too, if this one didn't work out.

I phoned the facility and asked to speak to admissions.

"First of all," I said, "thank you for responding so quickly to my questions. I do have a few things I need clarified. What about haircuts or his nails?"

"Every Thursday," he said, "we have someone who does haircuts and a podiatrist comes one to two times per week."

"What about phone calls? My dad won't let us get him a phone and he can't stand in the hallway like he has to do now."

"All rooms have their own telephones."

"What kinds of outings do you take, or what activities are offered?"

"Movies, karaoke, we've gone to the Shedd Aquarium, the zoo, places to enjoy nature."

"When we come to visit, is there a room we can go to spend time with him?"

"Yes, there's a large garden patio with a waterfall fountain. Inside, there's a private dining room the family can reserve. There's an activity room. There's also a beautiful library and lounge with couches and a piano."

Okay. He had me at 'piano.'

I updated Jackie.

"So, once I get those two documents, social security award letter and a referral letter, from his current facility," I said, "and when Dad agrees to do so, and when they have a decent bed available, we can move him over."

"How much will it cost?" she asked.

"Because of the money in his bank account, he might have to enter as a private pay. For a semi private room, it's $11,000 a month."

"That's a lot of money. Do we have enough for that?"

"No, not really, but they said they have social workers there who can handle all the Medicaid and insurance for free. They seem to be under the opinion that we should have him enter as a private pay with a pending status rather than remove him entirely from Medicaid."

"How can they charge so much to put him in a room with three other people?"

"I don't know. When I researched it, most places charge over $10,000 per month."

"That's ridiculous."

"Agreed."

Considering the physical condition and short-staffing at a lot of these places, I knew the corporate owners must have been making a lot of money. I wondered why couldn't society cap the profits at these facilities? Perhaps that would encourage them to pay their staff more and take better care of patients and the building itself and offer more services.

"What about the attorneys?" Jackie asked. "Aren't they figuring all this out?"

"I just signed the retainer agreement with them, but it's been tough finding the time to talk during all of the holidays. We tentatively scheduled a phone appointment for the first week of January."

"I hope they get you some answers soon. This is too much stress for you to deal with."

I appreciated that she acknowledged that. Sometimes it felt so isolating to be the sole person who cared for or coordinated the care of a loved one while everyone else could ignore the problem and go on with their everyday lives. This was the case with us: I did everything because Jackie so often viewed the situation as too stressful for her to deal with. Sometimes a few words of comfort and a thank you went much further than you'd think in keeping someone from breaking apart under stress.

Jackie and I both knew there weren't enough funds remaining in the trust to pay for more than a few months of his care. We preferred not to run out of money completely so that we could continue to meet his needs with any additional items such as clothing. I didn't have any idea what we'd do if we ran out of money; None of us—Jackie, Keith, or I—had any extra disposable income to pay towards Dad's care. We were all barely getting by as it was.

With Christmas approaching, my siblings and I sent Dad and the staff each another box of See's chocolates—a gift we could afford and one which provided some level, even if short-lived, of emotional comfort and joy. At least Dad would have something to look forward to until we could get him moved, hopefully in early 2020.

Until I talked to the attorney, all I could do was wait.

CHAPTER FORTY-ONE

Dress Shopping

On JANUARY 2, 2020, I perused the racks in the bridal shop, taking pictures of price tags with item numbers to select wedding dresses to try on. Sparkling sequins, smooth satin, gorgeous lace, V-neck, scoop neck, train, no train, A-line, princess cut, ballroom, white, cream, champagne, so many options.

This was my third time at this store and after trying on more than a dozen dresses, I still hadn't found the dress. For a purchase that was easily going to exceed six or seven hundred dollars, I wanted to at least feel good in what I'd be walking down the aisle in.

I glanced at my phone. At one o'clock, I had an appointment to speak with the Medicaid attorney, Jill. But it was already after one. I had lost track of time.

I sent a quick email on my phone and got back a response that she'd call me in a couple minutes. I had hoped to make it back to my car to take the call, but unfortunately, I didn't get the chance. So, I paced a corner of the bridal store and kept out of earshot from other patrons and employees.

"The first thing we need to do," Jill said, "is to figure out how much money the state paid for your father's care while he's been at the facility. If he had funds, Medicaid shouldn't have been paying."

"How do I get that info?"

"See if the facility can get that information for you. Otherwise, we'll have to try to go through the state, which can take longer."

"How much longer?" I turned to walk in another direction to avoid a mom and daughter heading to the dresses by my side. "We're trying to get him moved into a new facility, hopefully next month, or at least by March. But this whole situation is a problem. What do we do?"

"After we figure out how much was paid on his behalf, then we can make some decisions. If you have enough money, then you write the state a check to reimburse them. If you have more than enough, we'll figure out how you can do a spend-down to get his assets down below the limit. There are allowable expenses like pre-paid funeral expenses. If you don't have enough, we'll have to settle with them."

Bleh. I was here looking at wedding dresses and she was talking about my dad's funeral.

"Will he get dropped from Medicaid and… and…" I paused while an employee approached me to restock a bulky gown on the rack behind me. When she left, I lowered my voice. "And if so, how do we pay for his bills to keep him in the facility? It's extremely important to us that he doesn't end up back on the streets."

"I understand. None of us want that to happen."

What didn't make sense was how difficult it was to get information as simple as "how much money do we owe you?" from his current facility. Neither Jill nor I had any luck throughout January.

Finally, a novel suggestion was made for me to contact an Illinois State Senator, explain the situation, and see if they could be of help. The assistant who took down my information was just as surprised as I was that it was so difficult to find a way to pay back the government. They agreed to intervene on our behalf. If the issue wasn't resolved by the end of February, they told me to call them back and we'd come up with a new game plan.

Sometimes allies come from the most unexpected of places. I would've never thought of contacting a senator for this. But when a person feels stuck without knowing what to do next, the best thing to do is reach out in every direction and ask for help.

CHAPTER FORTY-TWO

MAKING PLANS

I LIKE PATTERNS. I always have. A big one was approaching: 2-20-2020.

"I know our wedding with our family and friends is in June," I said to Leo, "but what if we get legally married first at a small ceremony at the historic courthouse in Santa Ana? Just you, me, and the boys."

"You don't want to wait?" Leo asked.

"I know how bad you are at remembering dates." I jabbed him in the side playfully. "How could either of us ever forget our anniversary if it was two, twenty, twenty-twenty? We can make an appointment for 2 PM."

"Not 2:20?" He laughed.

"I have to do a practice run with the hair and makeup for the real wedding, so why not do it the morning of February 20?"

So, our plans evolved in that way. I picked out a simple above-the-knee white dress with a lace-flowered pattern—something I could wear again. I also broke down and bought a similar, simple full-length dress and a crystal studded belt; both dresses were comfortable stretch lace. I figured that if I couldn't find a gown I loved before June, at least I wouldn't walk down the aisle naked.

Because our three boys didn't have their suits, and Leo hadn't yet gotten his tuxedo, we picked out the nicest dress shirts each of the three boys had.

"I want to hire a photographer," I said.

"Why spend the extra money? We hired one for our June wedding."

"It won't cost that much and I want to have some nice pictures."

After more prodding, Leo relented.

Even though we had my engagement ring, which would become my wedding ring, Leo needed one, and no, I wasn't going to let him wear a rubber wedding band as he suggested.

At our local jeweler, we found him a gorgeous ring being sold on consignment—a thick gold band with a double row of diamonds along the front. And it fit perfectly. It was meant to be.

Leo's son Chris would meet us at the house in the late morning that day, and we'd all drive over together in the afternoon.

A few days before our courthouse wedding, on Monday, February 17, Francine gave me some jarring news—she was no longer able to visit Dad or help with his care. Her husband was experiencing some health problems. Dad's case was handed over to another nurse, Amy, to visit with Dad. She had introduced Dad to Amy over a number of visits until he seemed comfortable enough with her.

Although I wasn't thrilled that he'd lose continuity of care, when I spoke with Amy, I was impressed by her genuine sense of care, so I was willing to give her a chance. Besides, what choice did I have?

One afternoon, while Leo and I were designing our centerpieces for our June wedding, I phoned Amy. Leo laid out round slabs of wood across the dining room table while I sorted through bunches of purple and pink silk peonies. I had time to chat while Leo delicately tried to ease white wooden table numbers into their bases.

"How is Dad doing?" I asked Amy. "We think we're getting pretty close to getting him moved. They received the paperwork and approved him. We're waiting for a bed to open up."

"Regarding your dad's thinking," Amy said, "he talked a lot about the mob being after him with Francine."

"Well, that's typical. He's probably not taking his meds." I opened a pack of silk greenery and divided them into twelve tin vases, eight for the wedding tables for our guests and a few extra for decoration.

"He brought that up with me Monday but said he didn't want to 'put me in danger.' When we were out, he was very talkative and the content was about his past, and current, abilities to see angels and demons and he told me a few 'experiences' he had while he was on the streets. There seems to be a religious preoccupation with all of this."

I briefly filled her in on some of Dad's history as a "self-proclaimed prophet of God" who traveled the world before he disappeared and described my book.

"Sounds fascinating. I'll have to order the book," she said. "I understand his mental health condition has been chronic and so I wonder if he's been without delusional thinking recently. He's on an antipsychotic and takes it regularly per the staff."

Leo nudged me. He held out three different colors of ribbons. "Which one for the vases?" he whispered. "I'll cut them up."

I pointed to thick, dark purple. "That's news to me," I said to Amy. "I thought he was refusing."

"I discussed the meds and his thinking with him and actually asked if it helps his visions or any voices quiet down and he said it does. It sounds like he's never without them though."

"I'm shocked he allowed you to discuss that. He bristles at talk of schizophrenia." I opened another pack of silk peonies and divided those into the vases.

"I didn't use that word. When we talk about what he wants in terms of living, he sounds rational. Francine said he has come a long way in terms of talking about anything with us so we are making positive moves developing trust with him."

"The new place does take Medicaid but I'd wait until he goes and if they accept him. I told him I think it's a step up. Maybe they can get him out of bed to distract him from the voices and visions."

"He needs encouragement and activities but it seems he doesn't get much of either where he is," Amy said. "He has declined to accept the relationship between lying in bed all day and not sleeping at night. We're going to have to work on that."

Great. He feared the Mob again. Just when we'd been making so much progress. But maybe it was just the switch to Amy that triggered that. I hoped that after everything settled down again, we could resume his progress. And maybe, just maybe, he'd be able to attend my wedding, or at the very least, write a congratulatory speech she could record which I could play at my wedding.

CHAPTER FORTY-THREE

All That Glitters Isn't Gold

WEDNESDAY, FEBRUARY 19, 2020

"Amanda, listen," Dad said at the beginning of the phone call he'd initiated. "I'm telling you that you need to read it and believe it with all your heart if you want to be saved."

I shook my head and ground my teeth. "Dad—"

"Forget about everything else in this world. Focus on the next. It's the only—"

"Dad, I know. You've told me before. You sent me a Bible and—"

"Do you still have it?"

"Yes, but, Dad—"

"There is no 'but.' I know these things. Daddy knows. You listen to me."

"Come on, we've been—"

"You must be baptized, a full body immersion, and accept Jesus Christ as—"

"Dad, stop. Just stop. Please. I know. You've already told me all this before."

He paused. "But you're not listening."

My heart was racing and my cheeks were hot. I tried to slow my breathing. Why is he doing this again? He was back to his old ways. "Can we talk about something else?"

"God has spoken to me. I've had visions. You don't believe me, but I know these things."

I sighed loudly. "Dad, I've got to go. Can I call you back?" I didn't have time for this bullshit today. Not with me getting married tomorrow.

"Don't be so stubborn," he said.

"I love you, Dad. I'll talk to you soon."

We ended the call. I closed my eyes and rested my head in my hand.

How soon could we get Dad moved? I couldn't deal with a repeat from the past.

I sat and typed an irritated email addressed to Francine, Amy, and Melody. Before I sent it, I reread it and revised it a couple of times, after I had a chance to collect my thoughts and not cry or scream at the screen.

> I am pretty concerned about my dad's degrading mental health. Today he phoned me and gave me the same religious speech that he used to give me during all the years he was experiencing the most psychosis and paranoia.
>
> This is significant because he has not given me this bizarre religious advice for the last year since I reconnected with him, with the exception of when he had the heart attack and I was there in the hospital with him, which of course is when he was under a tremendous emotional strain.
>
> I started getting concerned when Amy said he was feared the mob was after him and Francine. That's also a sign that he's going downhill fast.
>
> I've been so hopeful these past twelve months. He's actually been the most normal "old dad" I've seen since he first got sick in 1996. There was very little sign of that mental stability today on the phone call.
>
> Is he on the same medications? Is he sleeping? When he starts getting delusional, he used to fake out the nurses and spit out the

> medicine or pretend to take it. At that point he only got worse and worse because he wasn't really on the medicines.
>
> Please advise on what we should do.

Because as much as I'd gone through with him, and as much as I'd learned over the years, I once again was at a loss of what to do. His recovery was a mirage, an imaginary carrot dangling in front of my face. Fuck this.

I relayed the information to Jackie and Keith. Jackie didn't have any idea what to do.

"Well, what did you expect?" Keith said. "Nothing's changed."

Perhaps Keith was right. The circle continued. It was like the cycle of abuse; I'd been wooed during the honeymoon phase before his irrationality and mental instability broke through and lashed me again.

Was I ready and willing to get through another cycle with him again?

I laughed, because, once again, it was laugh or cry.

Let's hop back on the Merry-Go-Round and go along for the fucking ride. Just enjoy the pretty sparkles when the light hits them just right. It was better that I at least remembered not to be fooled by his progress, because the glitter wasn't gold.

And in the meantime, I needed to dry my tears and get ready for the big day.

CHAPTER FORTY-FOUR

2-20-2020

Despite the troubling phone call with Dad, I had to clear my mind to get ready for the wedding the next day.

Late at night, I turned to Leo. "Babe? We forgot something."

"What?" he asked as he laid out his suit.

"A bouquet."

"Do you need one?"

"I want one."

"Where are we going to get something like that, this late at night?"

So, there we stood in front of a mostly empty flower section in the grocery store. The sad bouquets of roses had some wilted buds. Some of the lilies were dried with spent blooms hanging at the end. A few other lonely flowers stood in the black plastic bins along the wall.

I looked at him. He had a bouquet of mostly open white roses.

"Awesome." I smiled. "Let's buy several of what's left and piece something together."

So that's what we did. We used some burlap ribbon and some ends of purple ribbons we had from the purple and pink peony centerpieces Leo had been hot glue-gunning together—see, I did mention he's a unicorn, right?

He cut them and I arranged greenery around the edges, and pretty soon we had a beautiful bouquet with white and red roses and purple flowers. I gave him a kiss on the cheek.

"I love it," I said. "Thank you for your help."

"Glad you're happy." He smirked. "By the way, I'm not wearing a tie."

I rolled my eyes, but was too tired from the day to argue. Dad's phone call had gotten under my skin. I needed to focus on the wedding at hand.

The morning of the twentieth, while I sat in the chair at the hair salon, watching in the mirror as my stylist hair-sprayed the wispy curls she'd created, I realized I didn't want Leo to see me until we got to the courthouse. Call me old-fashioned or superstitious, but it didn't feel right.

I texted a friend, who I knew stayed home with her kids most days and worked part-time, on the off-chance she was available.

"How exciting!" She squealed. "Yes, I'm home. I'll make myself available. Head over to my house and I'll drive you there."

"And be our witness?" I asked.

"You betcha."

I loved every minute of that day. We took fun photos at her house before we left.

My friend and I arrived first. We beat Leo there and he was a few minutes later than our agreed upon meeting time, a significant fact in our world, because that was probably the first and last time that I could claim to be early. Usually, my M.O. was to be overly optimistic about the time, which resulted in me being late.

At least for the rest of our lives, whenever Leo sat in the living room tapping his foot, waiting for me to be ready to walk out the door, I could remind him, "At least I got to the courthouse before you for our wedding."

"It was the boys' fault," he said.

Didn't matter.

The photographer snapped photos of the moment Leo and our sons walked through the door. He captured the expression of admiration when Leo first saw me, us on the historic staircase, the moments leading up to our "I do," and us all in a row holding up fingers to form the numbers 2-20-20. And much to my surprise, my friend, who held my purse and phone for me, filmed the entire ceremony, complete with both Leo and I getting choked up while reciting our vows in the chapel room under the fake flower arch.

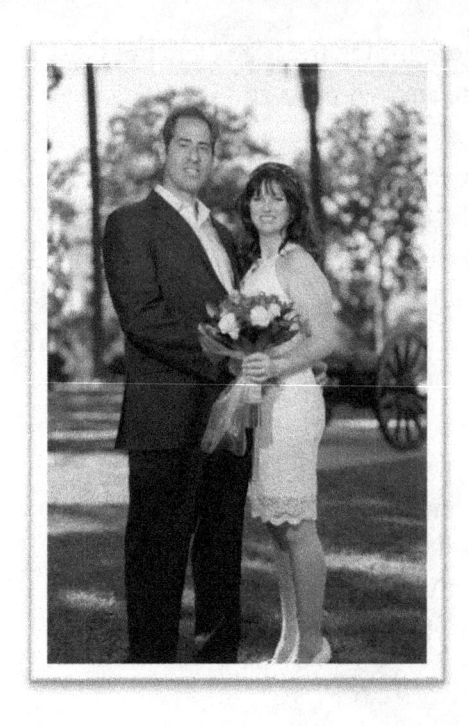

Afterward, our newly joined family got in the car to head over to Cheesecake Factory to celebrate. On the way there, I texted and emailed photos and videos to our friends and family.

When I refreshed my email, one appeared from my attorney Jill. Even though today's focus was on my courthouse wedding, SMI doesn't respect dates and events, and important details had to be attended to right away.

Because I'd had no luck finding out the total amount Medicaid paid for Dad's medical care, Jill had been trying to get that information from the Illinois Department of Healthcare and Family Services. Jill wrote:

> Dealing with these offices has been particularly ridiculous. I finally did speak to someone who seemed fairly knowledgeable on how to resolve overpayments. However, when I suggested reducing the amount owed, he referred me to his supervisor.... Who turned out to be the guy I've been communicating with for weeks who has NO IDEA what is happening. He barely seems to know where he works.
>
> Regarding the past payments, I was misreading the ledger. The actual amount owed is $86,000. My expectation is that they are now sending me a formal letter requesting payment with instructions on how to make that payment. If you would like me to counter with a lesser amount, I will do so, however I am doubtful that anyone involved is going to have the authority to negotiate this.

I jotted off a quick reply to all that we needed to move forward in making the payment as soon as we received the letter. I couldn't waste any additional time trying to negotiate something that could be impossible to negotiate. I needed Dad to get moved into a new facility.

Then I joined my newly combined family, my husband Leo, my two sons, and my now stepson, in the restaurant booth. I raised a glass of wine and sunk my teeth into some peanut butter and caramel fudge swirled cheesecake, and tried my best to forget about Dad.

When we all arrived home, on our doorstep we found a card, a box of chocolates, a bottle of champagne, and flowers from my friend.

Life could be wonderful and that was one of those moments.

CHAPTER FORTY-FIVE

The Move

MONDAY, FEBRUARY 24, 2020

I allowed myself a break from the dad drama for a few days. Then I sent Amy an email, and as I had been doing lately, I cc'd her boss Francine, Melody from the trust company, and Jill from the law office.

> Hi Amy, what did Dad think of the other place? Where and when are we moving him? It's been a busy last couple weeks for me. I got married this past Thursday. I told Dad on the phone. I'm going to check in with him tomorrow to see if he got the invitation for my June ceremony. I know of course that he can't go, but I wanted to send him one so he feels included.

The next day she responded:

> Hi Amanda, Today I took your dad to visit the new place, which he liked. Hopefully they'll accept him. The staff there is great at getting residents to activities. He complained a lot today about feeling weak. I'm sure it's not helpful that he spends so much time in bed. He mentioned he's used a walker in the past. I wonder if he can get a PT eval for one now although he doesn't walk very much. He didn't complain as much when we had our last tour.

On Tuesday, March 3, 2020, I got a voicemail from Chicago with even more great news: the new, much-improved facility had accepted Dad's application now that a bed opened up, and would be looking into setting up the transfer. Dad would finally get to enjoy the outdoors every day if he wanted to on the garden patio where he could listen to the waterfall and birds under the trees.

With his voice croaky and shaky, Dad left me a voicemail. "Hi Amanda, there's a new facility. I wanted to let you know they may move me. Can you call Amy?"

Perhaps Dad was looking forward to the move? I could hope. Either way, at least he was involved in the decision making.

Sometimes it seemed like a lot of news hits on the same day. I got an email with attachments from our attorney, Jill. Apparently, after I had spoken to the senator's office, the Illinois Department of Healthcare and Family Services finally sent a letter with directions on where to mail a check, as well as the pages of financial records showing the amount due was $84,826.48. The letter was signed by an individual in the Liens and Estates Unit in the Technical Recovery Section. With a specific department that specialized in recovering money, I wondered why it had been so challenging for them to get the information to Jill.

At any rate, this meant that, after paying the attorney fees, setting aside the money for the pre-paid funeral expenses, and reimbursing the state for Medicaid expenses, Dad's Citibank account should be under the two-thousand-dollar threshold.

I immediately wrote out the check and sent it along with a copy of the letter and documentation to the address listed. I was sure that would be a check they'd deposit immediately. It wasn't every day that someone called up the government and offered to give them back nearly a hundred thousand dollars without being asked to do so.

But it was not only the legal thing to do, but the ethically and morally correct course of action. Keith and Jackie absolutely agreed with me.

Some people seem to distort the truth or point out unrelated inequities or inefficiencies to find justification for doing the wrong thing. This has become apparent to me in the months and years after I wrote that check.

Oftentimes, when recounting my experiences and retelling this story, I encountered slack jaws and wide eyes.

"Have you lost your mind?" one of our friends said to me. "That's the stupidest thing I've heard of. They didn't know about the money, so why on Earth did you give it to them?"

"Taxpayers had paid for my dad's care under the assumption that he was financially in need. The money should go towards the care of another individual who needs it."

"You wrote a check to the government for a hundred thousand dollars?"

"It's legally what needed to happen. Besides," I said, "it was only eighty-five thousand."

He shook his head. "You're a good person, I guess. Not many people would do that."

These reactions made me wonder: why didn't everyone else have the same code of ethics, especially the ones who purported to live their lives according to the Bible or another religion whereby they answered to a higher God. Even Mary and Joseph paid their taxes.

The next day, Wednesday, March 4, I answered the phone and a man who identified himself as a patient coordinator at the new facility said, "We're moving your dad here at 6PM tonight. Regarding the therapy you asked about, we're going to be starting him out with intensive physical and occupational therapy for up to two hours a day. He'll be in good hands here."

"Excellent. As soon as possible, I'd like to meet with his entire care team in person." I had learned the terminology, what our rights were, and what I could ask for. I had also learned it was far more effective to meet everyone face-to-face. Better results that way. "I would like everyone to be there: his psychiatrist, primary doctor, physical therapist, coordinators, everyone."

"Understood. When would you like to schedule that?"

"As a teacher, it's hard to take time off, so I can fly out during my spring break in April."

I talked to Leo and confirmed he'd still be available to travel with me. My husband, no longer my fiancé, would finally get to meet my dad.

Once Dad was safely in a much-improved living space, I planned my trip to Chicago. I booked two flights to O'Hare. We'd fly home the day before Easter. I booked a room at The Westin on Michigan Avenue, and our rental car at O'Hare—always book in advance!

I couldn't wait to introduce Leo to my dad. The old dad would have loved Leo and be thrilled to have him as a son-in-law. I hoped the new dad at least liked him and trusted him well enough to converse with him.

And everything was as great as it could be… until it wasn't.

CHAPTER FORTY-SIX

The World Shuts Down

There are certain days in a generation's lifetime that start out with "Do you remember where you were when…?" followed by some unmistakable horror—the bombing at Pearl Harbor, JFK's assassination, MLK Jr.'s assassination, the fall of the USSR, the Twin Towers on 9/11, and now, for the newest generation, add: Covid-19 and insert the day where your life changed—whether it was the date of a job loss, a school closure, a family member becoming horribly ill, or worse, the death of a neighbor, a friend, a loved one.

Normally, I read far more news from multiple outlets and sources than I should, bordering on unhealthy. Many people have not forgotten it was also the year of the word "unprecedented," with terms like fire tornadoes, fire lightning, and murder hornets. I wasn't doom-scrolling the news—I focused on quick updates about the court system, international politics, wars, local news, crimes. Okay, maybe a little bit like doom-scrolling. I call it staying informed.

I, like most Americans and many other world citizens, had never personally lived through a pandemic (Side note: Pandemic is a fun board game, but at that moment, it was too soon.).

Regardless, the political climate at the time was so divisive and depressing that I avoided spending too much time on the news. Instead, I diverted my attention to wedding planning—seating charts, signing contracts for the venders, and choosing cake flavors.

So, on Thursday, March 12, only a week after Dad's move, when I got the following voicemail from his new facility, I was perplexed:

"Hi, good morning, Amanda, this is Shannon from the facility and I'm calling to inform you that due to the current cases of coronavirus in the country, I'm really sorry to inform you that there'll be no visitors into the facility until further notice, and if anything changes, we'll surely give you a call back. If you have any further questions, you can call me back. Thank you and have a good one."

No visitors? Used to overreaction in the media with everything being labeled as "Breaking News!", I couldn't yet fathom the seriousness of the worldwide outbreak and the implications. I wasn't ready to cancel my trip to Chicago yet. Perhaps this was just an extra precaution because they had elderly people with compromised immune systems. Perhaps it was a temporary situation that would resolve itself before April. I decided I'd call her back the next day.

But on Friday, March 13, another layer of reality presented itself. That was the day I got sent home from work, the day our schools closed in-person learning. The abrupt announcement came over the intercom, that students needed to clear their lockers and leave campus, while staff were to report to the auditorium for an urgent meeting. Because of my break from following the news, I hadn't read much about the coronavirus.

For me, the words thrown out didn't make much sense in a high school setting—*distance learning, Zoom, online class*. We'd need to attend meetings over Zoom and approve a new online schedule and work within our teacher teams to modify instruction to deliver content remotely.

"With no notice? Maybe this will just be for a week or two." That's what I naively said to the science teacher as we walked back out to the parking lot.

"Worst case," I said, "We'll be back after Spring Break."

He shook his head and said, "Nope. We're not coming back this school year. They're canceling sports games, too. Trust me, this is more serious than people realize. You'll see."

I thought he was overreacting, but then again, he understood science. I did not.

Immediately my phone blew up with messages from everyone who got the same news from every walk of life, and not just in California—the world was shutting down.

I realized there had been strange hints leading up to that moment: seeing my students, most of whom were Asian, coming to school with masks, starting around January. It started with a couple, then a few more, and then enough of them to make me wonder why. I hadn't stopped to consider that in Asia, many of their family members may have already gone through something similar, the H1N1 bird flu, and unlike the rest of us, were far more prepared to deal with it.

I thought of Ebola outbreaks in Africa. The Black Death, bubonic plague, in Europe during the Dark Ages in the 1300s. The Spanish Flu here in the United States from 1918-1920. That was the extent of my historical knowledge of anything on a similar scale.

All of that was so far removed from my life that I didn't see the signs that something was amiss here at home until it was too late to prepare for the changes. I felt somehow insulated from the problems that happened over there.

I considered how different our lives were now compared to 1920: international travel could spread diseases from one tiny town to anywhere in the world within hours, exponentially, thanks to the magic of modern transportation.

So many thoughts flooded my mind—Leo and I had already put down deposits for our June wedding—the venue, photographer, videographer, and more. Our honeymoon to the Dominican Republic scheduled for July had been paid in full.

We couldn't deal with any of that, yet.

Leo and I sat down that evening to add an entry to our daily journal. It was a serendipitous gift I had gotten for us for Christmas in 2018. On January 1, 2019 we started this three-year journal for couples that provoked discussion with a different prompt every day—the next two years' answers would be recorded below the previous, so that on each page, we could see how our answers to the prompts changed over three years.

We had no idea when we began the book that it would document our lives through engagement, marriage, Covid-19, and more.

On March 13, the prompt was: "I hate having to _____."

Leo wrote, "do status reports for work," while I wrote "start teaching remotely (online)."

For the next couple weeks, I was preoccupied with my new reality and scrambled to figure out the technology needed to teach from home. One afternoon, after teaching a virtual class, I checked my voicemail. Dad had left me a short message, said with a tinge of sadness, "This is Dad phoning you but I guess you're on another call now, so I'm here. Bye."

I tried to stay in contact with Dad, but life for him became harder because he was supposed to stay in his room. I wondered whether getting him moved was a good or bad thing.

But when I started checking the online databases reporting the stats for nursing homes, I knew how very fortunate we were. The number of patients getting, and dying from, Covid-19 was far higher, every single week, in his previous facility.

So, maybe, just maybe, the move had saved his life.

Checking the weekly updates in the local newspaper that charted the number of cases locally, by state, and by country, as well as the number of deaths, became a part of my routine. So did watching the bell curve rise sharply with no downward curve in sight. And talking to my friend, an ER nurse at a hospital who relayed horror stories from the Covid unit, and the deaths—this was unlike anything she'd ever seen. And hearing from friends whose neighbors—middle-aged people like me—had died. And, no, not all had had pre-existing conditions.

And then speaking with others who personally knew no one who had been hospitalized or died from the virus and expressed skepticism that they were being sold on a false narrative, fake news, that Americans were making a big deal out of nothing, that Covid was nothing worse than the flu.

But this wasn't just happening to America—it was happening to the world.

I believe most people and governments did the best they could with the lockdowns, social distancing, and mask mandates based on the information they had. I just wished there wasn't so much fighting over it. The fear and anger from both sides seemed to be as contagious as the virus.

Unlike an enemy invader from another country, this viral enemy was invisible and pervasive. Because it's hard to fight something you can't see, I felt it best to be cautious and avoided being around others.

It seemed disingenuous to blame one side or the other for their best guesses on how to handle the pandemic and instead to move forward with the lessons learned—all while realizing that each virus is unique and the next pandemic, whenever that may be, could require a completely different response.

As for the current situation, though, I remained worried for myself, my family, especially my mom, my dad, and, in particular, Hilda. I couldn't get a hold of her.

I'd reached out to her several times through Facebook Messenger, but my text messages, audio calls, and video calls went unanswered. Not knowing what had happened, my mind ran through various scenarios of all the rotten possibilities. I hoped she was safe, but I couldn't know for sure.

It left me with an uneasy feeling.

CHAPTER FORTY-SEVEN

Covid-19

MARCH 27, 2020

I held out hope for as long as I reasonably could that Covid-19 and the related restrictions would pass quickly. But no, I watched the case count and death rate tick up at the nursing homes, especially Dad's former facility.

I resigned myself to reality and canceled the plane tickets, rental car, and hotel. It was clear we weren't going to Chicago anytime soon. In the meantime, I phoned Dad as often as I could. I couldn't imagine how the instability would affect his precarious mental health. Getting moved, new roommates, new traveling nurse—first Francine then Amy—and now no more spending time with Amy because even she wasn't permitted to visit.

Additionally, what troubled me was that as of April 15, the state of Illinois still hadn't cashed the check for eighty-four thousand dollars. I contacted my attorney.

"They haven't cashed it?" Jill said. "Are you kidding me?"

"No," I said. "Citibank would have notified me because their fraud department notifies me every time one of your checks goes through because they are so large."

"I'll email the guy. So absolutely ridiculous! The State is burning through money, they should cash every check they get!"

I contacted the Illinois Senator's office again as well.

Miraculously, on April 17, the check was deposited. The phrase "the squeaky wheel gets the grease" came to mind. But boy, did we have to do a lot of squeaking.

From one financial issue to another, I discovered Dad's social security payments still hadn't been transferred over to the new facility. I emailed Leslie, Jill's assistant who was now handling the Medicare end of things, for guidance, and messaged one of my contacts at Dad's new facility. The woman from his nursing home informed us that Social Security was closed during the shutdown, and because they submitted additional paperwork just after the April 15 cutoff date, they wouldn't start receiving his Social Security checks until May.

I found it slightly amusing that it was easier to work with the Social Security agency during the 2020 shutdown than to deal with Dad's bank and pension company during 2019.

While at home teaching, I had more flexibility to do things like eat lunch and use the restroom. Leo ran his meetings remotely and needed silence, so we kept the home office door shut. David had his earbuds in and did his schoolwork on one end of our dining table, while I taught at the other end.

Whenever I needed privacy to handle Dad's business, I hid out in my bedroom or in my backyard, which is where I had many conversations with, and about, Dad.

I frequently talked with Fred, Dad's nurse at the new place. Fred spoke clearly and kindly. I recognized his accent as Ghanian, like Priscilla's, the nurse who cared for my dad during his last heart surgery. In addition to Fred, I kept in close contact with Ashley, one of the social workers there, whose voice exuded warmth and positivity with a Chicago accent. Both became invaluable sources of information and communication. Unlike the last facility, there did not seem to be much turnover, an especially important fact during that time.

Covid-19 spread through Dad's facility. So much so that the entire second floor was redesignated for Covid patients only. On Monday, April 22, they reported twenty-nine cases and began the process of moving my dad, and any other healthy individuals up to the fifth floor.

"Amanda," Ashley said during a call, "we've been having a little bit of an issue with your dad. Can you have a talk with him?"

I stepped into my backyard. Even with a cool breeze, the sunshine burned hot against my skin, so I took a seat in the shade.

"What's he doing?" I was hoping he wasn't streaking naked through the hallways and punching people like I'd heard of others doing—the more people you meet who have loved ones with SMIs, the more stories you hear.

"Every time he wanders in the hallway," Ashley said, "I try to get him to go back to his room, because we need everyone to stay distanced. Well, he argues with me and tells me that he can't get sick."

"That's his delusions speaking."

"I know, but I'm trying to keep him healthy. I even put hand sanitizer in his hands which he doesn't really like. And he won't wear a mask in the hallway."

"He has nothing to keep him entertained because he doesn't watch TV. That may be because his vision isn't good enough to see it, but I don't know." I glanced over at hummingbirds fluttering around the orange flowers on my Birds of Paradise

"Unfortunately," Ashely said, "we aren't running activities right now, because of Covid."

"Understandable." The hummingbirds buzzed over to my water fountain and dipped their beaks and wingtips into the water. I wished I could tell Dad about them. "Can you also check to see if his phone is working because I've tried to call him many times and the only time that I've gotten through to him was when the nurse brought a cordless phone to his room. Now that doesn't matter since he's going to a different room. All of these moves are probably stressing him out quite a bit."

Several days later, while I was making scrambled eggs, I got another call from Ashley.

"Uh-oh," I said. "What did Dad do now?" I balanced the phone in the crook of my neck.

"We couldn't move him up to the fifth floor," Ashley said, "because he just developed a fever. So now he's back down on the second floor."

I set down the spatula and took the phone in my hand. "Is he okay?"

"Fred, his nurse, will phone you to give you an update as soon as we know more."

That wasn't the response I wanted. I turned off the stove and plated up food for David. I couldn't eat after that call, so I went in my bedroom and sent Jackie and Keith a message. We held our breath and waited.

"Amanda, this is Fred," the man with the Ghanian accent announced. His words came slow and deliberate. "I am calling to update you on your father. Good news… the fever is gone. But he has a cough. So, we are keeping him down here for now."

I thanked him, but immediately reached back out to Ashley.

"On Saturday when I talked to him," Ashley said, "he seemed quite out of breath and wouldn't talk. He answered yes or no questions and told me it was hard to breathe and he was exhausted."

"That's not good," I said. "Do you think it's Covid? How bad is it over there?"

"We currently have nearly forty cases."

"Out of a hundred and eighty beds? How many haven't made it?"

"There have been five deaths at this point."

I'd been checking the reported deaths from all the nursing homes in that area, and I knew most are significantly higher than theirs. "I'm appreciative he's there because your facility is be doing so much better than the others."

"We're doing the best we can."

"Even if Dad doesn't have a fever, that's not good if he's out of breath and coughing. How are the rest of his vitals?"

"I don't have that information with me."

On Friday, I got a hold of Fred again who checked his vitals: 95% oxygen and no fever.

"Your father is fine and doing all right," Fred said.

"But Ashley said he was out of breath."

"Maybe he's tired because he keeps going up and down the hallway in a wheelchair despite us constantly asking him to return to his room to reduce his exposure."

"He thinks, from his delusions, that the virus can't get him. I have not gone into great detail with him about Covid, but just told him that there is a virus which is why I had to cancel my flights out there in April."

It was frustrating, but not nearly as much so as for all of the other families who weren't able to hold the hand of their loved ones placed on ventilators, or taking their last breaths.

While Leo and I folded laundry on in our bedroom, I phoned Jackie to update her, but she didn't answer. I dialed Keith's number next.

"On the positive side," Keith said, "it sounds like he's getting exercise."

"Moving around in a wheelchair?" I asked.

"Well, he can work out his arms to prepare for a race with other patients."

"Very funny." I laughed. Leo threw me a quizzical look. "A few weeks ago, Dad used the word 'depressed' when telling me how he felt. I offered to send him photographs and he said that would only make him feel worse. I think he's pretty lonely."

"Understandable. Wouldn't you be?"

"I asked him if I could send him an iPad or some kind of device so he can see us and talk to us, but he absolutely refused." I put my socks in the drawer, all except the one without its match.

"Probably better than him reading news online. Would only make him more paranoid."

"Speaking of the news, I read that the employees at his facility are threatening to strike in two weeks."

"Well, I'm sure this situation isn't helping."

The next day, on May 3, I got a voicemail. Dad had tested positive for Covid-19.

CHAPTER FORTY-EIGHT

BELLIGERENCE

TUESDAY, MAY 5, 2020

Ashley's normally calm, measured demeanor was clearly replaced by agitation and frustration when I heard her voice. "We don't know what to do with your dad."

I hurried over to my bedroom and shut the door. "What do you mean? What's wrong?"

"He's belligerent and yelling at the CNA's."

I heard screaming in the background. "Is that him?"

"Yes. He has Covid. We can't have him in the hallway. Sometimes you're able to calm him down. Could you?"

"I'll try."

"Joseph," Ashley turned on the sweet tone of voice. "Your daughter Amanda is on the phone. Can you—"

"No!" he shouted.

"She wants to talk to you… Can I give you the phone?"

"Hello?" His voice was croaky but angry.

"Dad?" I said. "I heard you're not feeling good."

"I feel terrible."

"Can you go back to your room?"

"No."

"Dad, you have Covid virus so you can't be in the—"

"I do not!" I heard a loud crash and screaming. In the distance, he yelled, "You're all a bunch of liars!" Then footsteps, someone was running.

"Amanda," Ashley sounded out of breath. "I'll call you back. Your dad just threw the phone at us."

I paced across the carpet and texted Keith and Jackie. She phoned me right away.

"What in the hell?" Jackie said. It sounded like she'd been crying. "So, Dad has—"

"I can't talk right now. The social worker is going to call me back."

"Call me," Jackie said.

I promised I would. I sat on my bed and stared at my phone, but I didn't have to wait long.

"We're thinking of possibly moving him into a psychiatric hospital," Ashley said. "We don't know what to do because we can't control him or redirect him. He will not go back into his room."

"Will a psych hospital even take him with Covid?" I asked. "Can't you give him a sedative or anti-anxiety medicine?"

"We tried. He refused the medicine and spit it out."

"Can you lie to him and tell him it's a vitamin?" I leaned back against my pillow and stared up at the ceiling.

"Normally, no, we aren't allowed to lie to patients."

"I'm the POA, so can't I instruct you to?"

"I doubt it, but I'll talk to the director and see if there's anything else we can try."

"I know he doesn't think he has the virus but how bad is it?" I asked.

"His oxygen is ninety-two to ninety-three percent."

"That's good, right?"

"That's only when he's on the oxygen. We'd like it to be above ninety-five. We don't want it to dip below eighty-nine. He's refusing the nose oxygen and takes it off every five minutes. They keep trying to put it back on him."

"So, if it does drop, does—" I was interrupted by a knocking on Ashley's end and hurried talking.

"Sorry," she said. "I have to go help them out there with him."

I took out my notebook, jotted down the medical details then immediately reached out to Amy and Francine. I advised them of the current crisis.

Francine took this one over and got back to me right away.

"I talked with Michael, the Director of Nursing." Francine said. "He reviewed the meds your father has been prescribed and offered several options to help him stay calm and accept the care he needs, including Haldol orally and as an injection, Ativan injection to help him stay calm—both are prescribed on an 'as needed' basis. He also has scheduled Olanzapine which he has been on for a while. Less is more and we hope that once Joseph calms, he will need less medication."

"But his behavior is worsening," I said. "And I'm worried because he has Covid."

"Fred said they're checking Joseph every four hours for cough, shortness of breath, temperature, and oxygen levels," Francine said. "He doesn't have other symptoms that are especially concerning."

"Not true. When I talked to Michael earlier and pushed him to give me the details, he did find on record that Dad has had a cough since April 29. I explained that Dad has been complaining he's short of breath and not feeling well. I told Michael that over the last week and a half, Dad keeps telling me that he's feeling worse and worse, which is why he's becoming so difficult and angry when they ask him to get out of the hallway and get back into his room."

"Interesting." She sighed. "I didn't know that."

"Michael said they'll keep monitoring Dad's oxygen, heart rate, blood pressure and respiration, but as of this point his vitals look stable. He said if Dad's oxygen dips below ninety-two percent while on the oxygen, or if his vitals take a turn for the worse, then they may move him out to the hospital. Apparently, I have to keep questioning them to get the entire truth and keep talking to my dad to see how he's feeling."

"We need to be careful that he doesn't get pneumonia."

"As someone who's dealt with pneumonia multiple times," I said, "I'm wondering if pneumonia is a risk to people with Covid, and if his oxygen levels are dipping, would it be better for him to be sitting up rather than lying flat on his back, so fluid doesn't settle into his lungs?" I had read that lying prone could help, too, but I didn't know how accurate the information was.

"You're a great advocate for your father. I'll send Michael the consent though they should have it in the file. Amy or I will follow up tomorrow. I wonder when the medical doctor last saw Joseph. I am so sorry we cannot visit."

"From a medical perspective, if Dad's got Covid pneumonia without a fever, will that show up in any of his vitals right now?" Suddenly, my head hurt. With all the talk of oxygen levels and breathing, my room felt suffocating. I dropped the notepad on my bed and headed outside to my porch swing.

"It should," Francine said. "Why?"

"The only way my doctor figured out I had pneumonia last year was by listening to my chest and doing an x-ray." I took a seat on my porch swing and squinted at the bright sun and blue skies. I thought back to my trip to Chicago with my sons and how I kept needing to rest on the benches. "I didn't have a fever or other symptoms, except for my extreme fatigue, which is only one of the things he's complaining about."

"I think we need to get the MD to weigh in," she said. "I'll call Michael in the morning. Amy may know the nurses there and may be able to get more or better information from them. We will certainly stay in touch with the facility and with you."

The next day, May 6, Amy gave me an update. Unfortunately, it wasn't good news.

CHAPTER FORTY-NINE

Pneumonia

WEDNESDAY, MAY 6, 2020

Amy had just spoken with the nurse practitioner who had been monitoring my dad.

"People can additionally have a superimposed bacterial pneumonia with Covid," Amy explained. "This is why they treat with antibiotics and he had azithromycin and Augmentin."

"What does that mean?" I pulled out my notebook and pen.

"Your dad's first chest x-ray showed symptoms which are called infiltrates and he had a fever. He was on oxygen because his levels were low 90's and on a physical exam he appeared to need supplemental oxygen. He may have been breathing heavily. That said, he wouldn't wear it. This has improved with the medications anyway and today his level is 99. She's ordered a repeat chest x-ray and the oxygen as needed."

"So, he's got pneumonia?" With my pen, I scribbled increasingly darker circles on the paper. I was pissed. "I told them so. Wait... you said a repeat x-ray? And he's already on antibiotics? Why didn't anyone tell me? With all the nurses I've been talking to over the last two weeks, nobody said anything to me about any of this."

"I really think everyone is overwhelmed," Amy said. "The good news is that he no longer has a fever, but he's still coughing and is refusing to wear a mask which would allow him to come out of his room. This is to protect him and the employees who are constantly coming and going… housekeeping, supplies, dietary etc. Being told to stay in his room is hard on him and I imagine they are frequently telling him to do so which is frustrating for everyone. I like to think they're patient but I'm sure it's very stressful. They have a lot of sick patients."

I slowed my breathing to calm down. "Yes, it sounds like they're taking good care of him. I'm just frustrated. I know Dad's frustrated. That's why they can't keep him out of the hallways."

"It's not helping that he's not consistently taking his psych meds and yesterday spit the pill out. That can account for his behavior, his low tolerance for being told to stay in his room."

I wasn't surprised. "This has been a long-term problem with him, the med refusal."

"I forgot to ask if they gave him an injection but I think they did and he is calmer. I asked if they can give him olanzapine in the disintegrating form called Zyprexa Zydis. We give it to people that we think may not be swallowing their meds, you can still spit it out but if it's in your mouth briefly it melts and voila… it's in."

I sat up to take notes and had her spell the name of the medicine. "How do we get him on this?"

"I'll ask the psychiatrist. If your father is not taking meds, they can discuss long-acting injections—"

"That's what I've asked for in the past. Why can't they do that?"

"Maybe in the future when his physical health is better and he's recovered. He can't have it now because of the crossover of side effects. That's just a suggestion if this problem persists. I sure hope things will get better. I give it often in the hospital but more so on younger patients. We often think less is more when it comes to medicating older adults."

"Right now, we need to focus on the pneumonia. Do you know when they are doing the next chest x-ray? I'd really appreciate it if the doctor would call me to give me the results of this 2nd x-ray. I want to know how it compares to the one they took before." I thought of all the news I'd been watching, the images of ventilators and doctors in isolation gowns and masks—personal protective equipment. The loved ones dying. "I don't want Dad to end up in the hospital and get worse." Tears welled in my eyes. "I don't want him to be alone."

Amy sighed. "I'm sorry I can't visit. It seems that I was just starting to get to know him, and him me. One of the things I've always liked about this facility is that the staff handles medical issues and doesn't get nervous or send people out to the hospital too quickly if they can be managed there. I agree the hospital can make things worse; they're not staffed to manage behavior issues on the medical floors. It would be unfamiliar to Joseph and I could imagine that if he got agitated, which may also be a possible symptom of hypoxemia, or wouldn't stay in his room, he would get quite medicated, which is not what we want."

"No, I just want him to get better."

"Me, too. I hope this is helpful and as reassuring as it can be considering the circumstances."

Each time I communicated with the staff at Dad's facility I kept track of how many liters of oxygen he needed and if that was going up or going down.

I phoned Amy. "I know he's probably not in any kind of urgent situation, but the whole idea of him having oxygen levels dropping, needing oxygen assistance, becoming very agitated—which has gotten worse each time I've talked to him over the last week and a half—more than nine days after having the fever, to me appears to be a decline in condition."

"It's really hard to force oxygen on people," Amy said. "That cannula is uncomfortable. But on that unit, they told me vitals are checked frequently."

"I hope the doctor is doing another x-ray soon." I thought of how sad Dad was when my sons and I left his side the last time. "I wonder if there's any way at all possible if somebody could show me a video of my dad or allow us to video chat for a minute or two."

"The Nurse Practitioner ordered the X-ray for today. I don't believe doctors are physically visiting but relying on the nurse practitioner and that is who you should call. She's there daily. I'm sure if you ask Ashley, she can

Skype with you. I've done this recently, too, and it made me feel better seeing someone."

I kept updating Jackie and Keith daily.

But on Thursday, May 7, I got news from the facility that Dad's condition had worsened.

I phoned Jackie.

"So," I said, "Dad wasn't on oxygen this morning and his level was up to ninety-five."

"That's good, right?" Jackie said. "That's what they wanted."

"Yeah, but now he dropped down to 92%, again, on the oxygen. Out of an overabundance of caution and actually Dad requested it, so you know he must be feeling crappy, he's going to be transferred to Weiss hospital today to get checked out. That's the same place where he had his heart surgery last year."

"That doesn't sound good."

Before they transported him, Ashley made it possible for me to video chat with Dad through Facetime on her personal cell phone. He was barely coherent. Although he was dressed, he had a full gray beard. He also was lying down the entire time, only opening his eyes briefly for a couple moments, and had a nasal cannula providing him with oxygen. He definitely looked like he needed to go to the hospital. I snapped a couple of screenshots, just in case... I shook off the thought.

A doctor from the Emergency Room phoned me a little while later.

"Joseph was down to 90/91% oxygen when he was admitted," he said. "Does he have a DNR?"

"Yes." Thankfully we had filled out the IDPD Uniform Practitioner Order for Life-Sustaining Treatment form, otherwise known as the POLST form, but more commonly referred to as a DNR, along with his POA docs. There were several sections, especially important for any person acting as a POA for their loved one.

On the form, under Section A, Cardiopulmonary Resuscitation (CPR), Dad chose "Do Not Attempt Resuscitation," hence the reference to DNR.

Under Section B for Medical Interventions, for when a patient is found with a pulse and/or is breathing, he chose "Selective Treatment: Primary goal of treating medical conditions with selected medical measures." This meant he was okay with IV fluids and IV medications, but specifically it states "Do Not Intubate. May consider less invasive airway support (e.g. CPAP, BiPAP)."

For Section C, Medically Administered Nutrition, he chose the last option: "No medically administered means of nutrition, including feeding tubes."

All of the above information was extremely important to know and would become increasingly critical in the future. What I wasn't prepared for were the detailed questions regarding Dad's DNR that the ER doctor next threw out at me. Most of it felt like medical jargon to me. He wanted specifics such as which interventions he could use like could he insert tubes going through Dad's leg, his arm, and specific medical procedures I'd never heard of.

I sent Francine an email asking for her help:

> I answered the best I could then confirmed my answers with Keith. I'm still waiting to hear back from Jackie. I told them yes to IV medication, yes to oxygen, yes to CPAP oxygen if needed and if he will permit them to do it, but no to the bigger IV that goes through his neck or his groin because I'm sure he will do more damage by ripping that out. And based on the POLST, I don't think he'd want that.

That same day, Amy and Francine, or perhaps Melody must have reached out to our attorney Jill, because Leslie, the Medicaid Consultant, contacted me. She pushed me to finish funeral pre-planning. This felt ominous. I was hearing that some Covid had been put on ventilators and because Dad would refuse that, perhaps it was time to make arrangements, just in case.

"This is a tough conversation," I said. "I'll try to determine what he wants."

CHAPTER FIFTY

The Plot

THURSDAY, MAY 7, 2020

Dad was not coherent enough to speak with me. Panicked, I didn't know what else to do. I got on a conference call with Keith and Jackie.

"I heard," Jackie said, "it's against Jewish tradition to be cremated."

"If we can't get word back from Dad regarding his preferences," Keith said, "which I don't know how I would ask that kind of question right now, then we should opt for a burial."

"Do either of you remember which cemetery Grandma and Grandpa are buried in?"

"Memorial Park in Skokie," Jackie said.

All three of us agreed we wanted Dad to be buried in the same place as his parents.

"I'll phone them now," I said. "And I'll reach out to Laurie because she's the one who made their funeral arrangements."

I tried not to dwell on the emotional aspects of this moment, pushing my feelings back for now. I went back into business mode. I had to get things taken care of. Now.

Before phoning the cemetery, I got in touch with Amy. I thought maybe she could help me figure out Dad's wishes. Maybe she had had this conversation with him.

"I've tried, too, to ask your dad end of life questions and never got anywhere," Amy said. "It can be a good idea to make arrangements when they are not needed so as to avoid this decision when you are in the middle of this difficult time. I have to say I'm not sure how things are being done with Covid."

"We want him at the same place as his parents, but we don't know what he would want. I think cremation may be against Jewish tradition."

"It depends how observant you are."

"None of us are. And especially not Dad who believed, and maybe still does, that he's a Christian prophet. But he was never religious at all."

"Well, hopefully you won't need this information, but there are Jewish people who choose cremation and are still at the Jewish section of the cemetery. I'm Jewish, my uncle was cremated as were other patients I've known or had."

I messaged Keith and Jackie again in our group text. Despite what Amy said, unless we heard otherwise from Dad, we'd choose burial. I contacted the cemetery.

"Melinda, what are our options?" I asked the Family Service Counselor.

"Call me Linda," she said. "And the Jewish section where your grandparents are buried is full. So, you have two options. There is space in another Jewish section, or there are plots available in a non-denominational section that's across the road from your grandparents."

"Really? How close?"

"I can take some pictures and send them to you today."

I forwarded the pics to Jackie and Keith.

"Look at the picture," I said. "The one where she circled where Grandma and Grandpa are and where this plot is."

"That's pretty close," Keith said.

"Yes, if you stood on his grave, you could see theirs."

"Then that's where we choose," Jackie said. "I think that's what they'd want."

Dad wasn't coherent enough to have this type of conversation. Besides which, who wants to ask their loved ones to make funeral plans while they're in the hospital? Nothing says give up, it's over, don't even bother trying to get better, like asking your family member, while they lay on a hospital bed on oxygen, "Hey, do you want to be cremated or should we buy you a coffin?"

I was hesitant to put a down payment and enter into a contract when I believed there was a good chance Dad would recover and we could ask him his wishes later on, when he was in better health. With all the news and horror stories of people dying from Covid, perhaps we were overreacting to this situation. Perhaps it was better to wait and see.

Fortunately, Weiss was able to stabilize Dad and discharge him back to the nursing home on Monday, May 11 after he spent most of the week in the hospital. I could only hope his behavior had improved. I swore he had nine lives. I just didn't know which one he was on at that point.

I tried to call him repeatedly, but couldn't get through. Either the phone in his room wasn't working, or he wasn't answering—either one was an equal possibility.

Finally, I reached out to Fred who told me Dad was doing well and was staying in his room pretty much. He brought the cordless phone to Dad.

I hoped he wouldn't throw it this time.

He wasn't very talkative. Both David and Justin got on the phone to at least say hi to him before he rushed us off. The only thing he wanted was to hang up.

I knew this wasn't just fatigue or Covid. Depression hung heavy on his every word.

CHAPTER FIFTY-ONE

The Distance Between

On, Sunday, May 17, 2020, I opened Facebook to see a friend request from Hilda, but it wasn't the same profile she'd been using before. I accepted the request and sent her a text through the Messenger app:

> How are you doing, Hilda? How is your family doing? Dad got COVID-19. Just to be overly cautious and careful, he went to the hospital for a couple days. He's doing so much better. He's back at the nursing home. Not to worry.

Unlike my previous overtures for the past few months, this time she responded:

> Hello? Everybody ok? Sorry to hear your daddy got the virus. Is he ok? Probably they caught on time, thanks to Lord he is better, here in most of the nursing homes older people die, is terrible, so far, I'm doing fine. Here by the beach no problem with the virus, but nobody can walk in the streets. Everyone has faces covered. The family is ok? Say hi and be safe. Love you all

I appreciated hearing from Hilda. The distance between her and us—Jackie, Keith, and me—had grown more than the miles that separated us.

But she still prayed for Dad and still loved us. This, especially in the midst of a pandemic, eased my worries and brought me comfort.

After checking in again with Ashley and Fred who assured me that other than his sadness, Dad was feeling better, I responded to Hilda:

> Yes, we're okay. Yes, Dad is okay. he does not like to stay in his room. I would get frustrated, too. We have to wear face masks, too. That's nice that you are at the beach house, not in the city. Are you allowed to walk on the beach now?

I didn't hear back from Hilda right away. But I did hear from Jackie.

"I'm really concerned that Dad isn't doing well," Jackie said. "I talked to him yesterday. He's very depressed."

"That's how he's been every day for the last month," I said. "I don't think it's anything to be concerned about at the moment." Again, there was my habit of trying to cheer her up rather than sit in an uncomfortable reality. But I couldn't fool her. Jackie was an empath, much more attuned to his mental state. Even when people hide sadness behind smiles, Jackie has an amazing ability to detect pain, connect with people at a deeper level, and make them feel safe enough to share the truth. Perhaps I was even a little jealous of the way she got Dad to share his feelings.

Honestly, I couldn't ever be as thoughtful as her, even if I tried. Whenever I confided in her that I was experiencing a difficult life event, she always lent an ear and oftentimes, I'd find a kind card with a moving message written in beautiful cursive inside my mailbox a few days later. I don't know if she realized how much I admired this about her. Instead of arguing with her, I should tell her more often. But again, this wasn't my strength—the whole feelings thing.

"He doesn't want to talk on the phone much," she said. "He sounds really sad."

"I offered to send him things like books or puzzles or electronic games to keep him busy, but he wants nothing. He won't watch TV, either. At least he's listening to them and staying in his room, so that's good."

"I fail to see how him staying in his room is improving his depression. Do you even care if he's sad?"

"That's a stupid question. Of course I care."

"Hmm." Jackie paused. "Well, obviously this conversation is annoying you, so I'll let you go."

She hung up. Even though it may have seemed I was dismissing her concerns, my intention was to ease her worries. When people hurt around me, I often find myself trying to distract them to relieve their suffering rather than to allow them to simply express their suffering. It hurts me to watch others hurt and out of this discomfort, I avoid getting too emotionally involved. But that doesn't mean I don't care.

Fortunately, Amy, even though she couldn't yet return to in-person visits, continued to help me coordinate Dad's care.

"Is there any way you can ask Dad's psychiatrist to adjust his meds?"

"Yes," Amy said. "I frequently see the doctor, but he's still doing tele-psych for the facility." She also worked as a nurse at another hospital, so we were fortunate for her other connections to doctors. "Last time I asked, he said your dad was stable, but I'm not sure that's true, maybe because he hasn't been able to see him. I'll talk to him again."

On Monday, May 25, another call came through from Chicago. It was Dad's nurse, Fred.

"We haven't been able to get your dad to take his medication since Friday."

"Can you mix it in his food?" I remembered how Hilda had tried that in the past.

"We tried to give it to him in some Ensure and ice cream and that worked but then on Monday he threw it away."

"His psych meds?"

"That and also his blood pressure medicine and aspirin. On top of that, we're having trouble getting him to stay in his room again. We had to redirect him at least ten times today. Can you talk to him?"

"I'll do my best." Realizing the last time that I asked him to do something, Dad threw the phone, I tried a different approach.

"Hey, Dad. How're you feeling?"

"Meh," he said.

"Do you remember your grandkids, David and Justin? They want to see you again soon." He didn't say anything, but at least he wasn't screaming, so I continued. "Remember all the trips you took us on when I was a kid? Remember the rain forest in Washington and you showed me the flying squirrel?"

"No."

"Well, I love squirrels and you showed me how those ones would spread open their limbs to leap from one tree to another. Do you remember that? Or the time you took us on all the cave tours and we learned the difference between the stalactites and stalagmites?"

"Maybe."

"I always forget which one grows up from the ground and which one grows from the roof of the cave. The guides used to tell us the cheesiest joke. When stalactites and stalagmites meet together, do you know what you call them?"

"No."

"A column. Get it?" He didn't laugh. "The doctor gave you the blood pressure medicine because of your heart attacks. Could you please take your medicine? I want you to be well so you can go out with us when we visit, like you did with Francine."

"I'll think about it."

That was better than no. I spoke with Ashley.

"Did he go back to his room?" I asked.

"For now," she said.

"Why can't he go into the hallways if he's over Covid? I know you're all doing the best you can and you're dealing with a lot of sick patients, but what if he's no longer symptomatic and can't give or get the disease, can't he then have a little freedom?"

"If your dad tests negative twice, then we can move him up to a floor with other recovered patients. Then at least he can go into the hallways with a mask. That would be better for him, and the staff."

On May 31, two weeks after my last message, Hilda responded:

> How is everybody? Still at home like in here? Is getting worse, people are tired, is terrible. I'm still here by the beach, I can't go back with my family, the good thing is here no sick people, is safe place. How is your dad? Is he ok? How you deal with his clothing,

they provide that? Is hard on you, are your sister or brother helping you? Is bad with this situation you can't travel pls let me know. Take care all of you, love you

When I wrote back, I omitted Dad's behavioral problems. I wanted her to remember my dad as the kind man she married, not the unreasonable, emotionally distraught one he was now.

Hilda, the restaurants are all closed indoors. You can only eat outside on their patios. The bars are all closed, too.

Dad was moved upstairs to the 5th floor because he doesn't have Covid anymore. He's doing okay but in a bad mood. Always tired. He doesn't want to talk on the phone for more than a few minutes. Jackie and I both sent him birthday cards. I wanted to send him Sees Chocolates but he said no.

Is it raining there? Are you able to go to the grocery stores? Sometimes they still run out of toilet paper, paper towels, and napkins. Is this happening there? I love you.

Love, Amandy.

Hilda and I went back and forth over the next few months, checking in with each other. I was relieved to have reconnected with her, and that she was able to communicate with Keith and Jackie, too, sometimes through video calls as well. She relayed how Covid was worsening in Argentina, and that everyone was isolated, same as it was in much of the United States. She sent more prayers and worried about my dad.

I worried about Hilda. Any hope she had of reuniting with my dad had basically been extinguished. How was she dealing with us finding Dad? Was it a reminder of her not being able to reconnect with him? I didn't want to upset Hilda, so, unlike Jackie, I didn't ask.

CHAPTER FIFTY-TWO

SEEKING ANSWERS

"Did you know that when they moved Dad up to the fifth floor," Jackie asked, "they stuck him in a room with three other people?"

"No," I said. "Someone should've called me. How did you find out?"

"Not easily. I thought he was only supposed to have one roommate. Is this a temporary thing?"

"I'll find out."

This wasn't the first time they had moved him after he'd recovered from Covid, but crowding him in a room with three others? The lack of communication was annoying. According to Amy, the fifth floor was for higher functioning patients so I wasn't sure how well that would go over.

"I've been hearing he still isn't medication compliant," Amy said. "So frustrating."

"Can't we get him on a long-acting injectable for his schizophrenia?" I asked.

"He's not a danger to himself or others and so it can't be forced."

"I wish they would. I couldn't imagine having to deal with a deluge of hallucinations and fear of enemies out to get me. It's not fair to him."

"We know he's so much better when he takes his meds but legally that's not a reason to do so by force, injections in particular. We can't even do that in the hospital. Only way to force meds that I'm familiar with is court and that's not an easy solution. You need a court order. Mental health court is notoriously strict as far as guidelines for this."

"But what if he's getting aggressive or causing the staff problems again?"

"I haven't seen him in person for quite some time so I can't provide personal opinion regarding his behavior. I've heard they're working on a plan for visits that may include them bringing the resident outside to a designated visiting spot. Last week I called and it's not official yet. Of course, the person needs to be willing to come out too. It's a start anyway."

"At least they've been helping me talk to him through FaceTime, so I can see him."

"Good. Oh, don't know if you heard, but his psychiatrist is moving out of state."

Awesome. More instability. Always fun starting all over again with a new provider. Back to square one.

On July 15, they moved Dad back down to the Covid floor because of a cough. He'd have to serve his new fourteen-day quarantine until July 29, even though his test and x-ray came back clear. They started giving him Claritin because he had a little bit of a runny nose, so maybe the cough was tied to allergies. I told them I didn't want him to keep getting moved back down because of a cough. It was frustrating.

I spoke with him on the phone. He didn't want to talk much because he said he was tired and resting. Once again, he did have a good long conversation with Jackie though.

On the bright side, we were able to have a discussion with our dad about end-of-life decisions. He indicated that he didn't have a preference, so we moved ahead with pre-purchasing one of the only two plots left in the section near our grandparents.

Even better than that, Amy was able to visit Dad in-person on August 18, and called me right after.

"I'm happy to tell you," Amy said, "I visited with your dad today. He looks good and was pleasant. He declined my offer to bring new clothes and shoes but I'll keep offering if you'd like me to. I will be going every other week and can stay involved and visit just let me know. The rules are to visit outside with masks for twenty to thirty minutes."

Perhaps the in-person attention would persuade him to resume his medication.

It didn't last long though. On September 2, he refused to see Amy, which didn't sound like him at all.

"I almost saw him," she said. "He said he'd visit but after thirty minutes coming down the elevator he apparently stepped out, turned around and said he felt he wasn't up to it. I'm not sure what happened but I'll keep trying. At least he initially wanted to."

My concerns increased when I finally got through the messed-up phone systems to talk to him on September 13. A nurse had to hold the phone for him so he could talk.

Dad sounded terrible. He sounded drugged and half alert. He said he was very weak and couldn't even get out of bed on his own anymore. He said they only exercise him downstairs once a week. He said he needed help to even get out of bed. He couldn't hear me very well so I also worried about his hearing.

Something was seriously wrong. Even when he had Covid, he was able to keep coming out of his room by himself on the wheelchair. I left a message for the social worker.

But then he completely changed only three days later, according to Amy's email:

> Hi Amanda, I saw your dad today and we had a nice long visit. He kept saying, "The weather is just right!" Overall, he was quiet but otherwise looked the same. I asked them to bring him in a wheelchair because the last time as you may recall he walked down and turned around. He says he uses his walker normally.
>
> There were no delusional references or discussion of fearing the mob and he looked relaxed. He says he takes his meds 'most of the time,' so I encouraged him to be consistent. I'll ask the staff too. He does admit to feeling down but wasn't very specific.

It didn't make any sense to me. It was as if there were two versions of my dad and none of us knew which version we'd get that day.

Granted it was a stressful time for everyone—by the end of October, Dad had been moved back to the Covid floor for the third or fourth time because of his coughing, sneezing, and respiratory symptoms, even though he didn't have a fever and he had already had Covid. It was frustrating because they did the labs and an x-ray but moved him before they got the results.

Even when he was back upstairs, hopefully for good, by mid-November, and accepting outdoor visits with Amy, another issue arose: during one of his long talks with Jackie, he expressed concerns again that he had Alzheimer's.

I relayed the message to Amy who could advocate on his behalf in person, but was told in-person visits had been suspended again because of an uptick in Covid cases.

"What specifics are making your dad worry about Alzheimer's?" she asked. "Have you noticed any changes regarding memory loss?"

"It's hard to say," I said. "Where do you draw the line between severe mental illness and Alzheimer's, or dementia?"

"I often think your dad lies down and ruminates about all the many things which worry him, some delusional like the mob following him, but not all. This isolation is making it so much worse. I'd hoped he would be more engaged. I'm not sure he will ever relax and not worry."

"Yes, but my sister and I have been asking for him to be checked for Alzheimer's because he's been expressing concerns since 2018 that he may have it. His memory is spotty. He told us his father had Alzheimer's and his mother had dementia. We are hoping they do an MRI brain scan."

"Please keep in mind that there is no medication for dementia and if he receives this diagnosis it may add to his depression. I don't think a neurologist visit would hurt but I'm not sure how much testing you want to do with this in mind. I'd just take it one step at a time. The facility is good about getting people out for scans and such should the doctor order it."

Which the doctor did. His MRI was scheduled for Wednesday, December 2.

Too bad they couldn't have used an MRI to diagnose his schizophrenia. Would there ever be a day when doctors could use routine tests to find evidence of a severe mental illness, to intervene before the condition worsened?

I hoped we'd get some answers from the scan.

CHAPTER FIFTY-THREE

The Results

On MONDAY, DECEMBER 14, 2020, Dad met with a neurologist, with Amy by his side. It was one of those important visits that he should've gone to with his wife or children. But because of distance and Covid and him having isolated himself from everyone, it simply wasn't possible.

I was teaching remotely fulltime and had to be available the entire school day, both for our two-hour block schedules with time for synchronized instruction in Zoom together with my class—videos on everyone, please, if possible, you can blur your background—and asynchronous practice time where I remained in Zoom for students to pop in and talk to me whenever they had any questions. The good part about all of that? David sat on the other end of the dining room table with his earbuds in attending his virtual school at the same time.

Sometimes he'd comment on my instruction while I was teaching just to make me laugh. Other times, he'd answer the jokes I offered to the students. I did enjoy having him nearby.

For my dad's appointment, I supposed I could've asked to be a part of the doctor visit via phone or video chat, but I felt it was more important to give Amy the ability to be fully present for my dad and the doctor, especially because she hadn't been able to see him in so long with all of the Covid restrictions.

I refreshed my computer screen waiting for word from Amy. What did the MRI reveal? Did Dad have Alzheimer's? I had heard there were drugs that could slow the progression of Alzheimer's with a proper diagnosis. What would the doctor say after reading the reports?

The MRI results shocked me. Amy wrote:

> Hi Amanda, Joseph just had his neurologist appt. I was able to spend a lot of time talking with your dad as the doctor was an hour late.
>
> Yesterday they told me they need to send him in a stretcher because when they put him in a wheelchair, he purposely slides himself down and is unsafe. I'm sure that sounds strange, but I see it quite often. It makes it difficult to evaluate his walking. I hear PT is trying, so we do need to give that a chance.
>
> The doctor did an exam and looked at the CT and MRI. Your dad has had many mini strokes. The location of strokes is in the part of the brain that controls motor function and explains why he complains that he feels off balance. It is also an explanation for memory impairment. Joseph tells me he feels confused but our conversation was good overall. He says, "I'm in bed a lot? I didn't realize that." He's already on a blood thinner which makes me think this isn't new information. These meds help prevent strokes.
>
> I also talked with the psych NP. Some of your dad's decline seems behavioral, for example, his unwillingness to feed himself, which he certainly can do. Covid keeps the residents in their rooms a lot and there's not much to do there. Isolation is not good for anyone's mood.
>
> He says he doesn't feel depressed but his symptoms are consistent with depression. He didn't reference any of the delusional thinking that I've seen in the past. Cognition and depression are intertwined. The psych said he may add Celexa and consider increasing his olanzapine.
>
> I suppose the question is what happens with this information?

Activity and physical therapy will help, but it's up to Joseph if he'll cooperate. This has been a barrier that he can't seem to overcome.

I haven't seen him in a while, but he looked better than I expected. I've always liked talking with him, he's always pleasant with me but has had a sad outlook on himself and his future. He often says it's hard to describe how he feels and will shrug his shoulders when I ask, how can we help you, but we don't want to give up on him.

I hope this isn't too discouraging but the reality is that neurological illness is chronic and progressive. Adding chronic psychiatric illness compounds symptoms. They can only hope to show progress if possible. Feel free to share your thoughts. It was nice to see him.

Stroke? Strokes? Plural. How? When? I remembered that my grandpa was a caretaker for my grandma after she suffered a stroke that affected her muscle control in half her face. Then, a massive stroke is what killed my grandpa. The news was heartbreaking.

Why was Dad having so many strokes? Jackie and Keith were as surprised and concerned as I was. None of us could comprehend. We needed more information.

"Amy, the strokes are news to us!" I said. We had no idea. I thought he was on blood thinners because of his three heart attacks. What does this mean?"

"When there are tiny strokes," Amy said, "the accumulation can result in memory impairment or what they call multi-infarct dementia."

"Do you think his condition and memory will improve, stabilize, or decline?"

"I've honestly never had the impression that his memory issue is so bad, but we only spend a few hours at the most together."

"He doesn't say anything when I remind him of places we've been or hikes we've taken."

"Well, he always strikes me as preoccupied with his thoughts and feeling hopeless which appear to affect his responsiveness. Being depressed makes one's memory 'foggy' and can make what's already a struggle worse."

"Was there also any sign of dementia or Alzheimer's in his brain scans?"

"Only the doctor can give this diagnosis and off the top of my head I can't say it's on his record exactly, but we discussed this as we looked at the scan reports."

"I hope he doesn't get worse. I want to visit him after Covid is over and hope that he will know who we are when we are there."

"I sure hope visiting will return with warmer weather and vaccines. I'm really an optimist, so I think it will be possible."

The staff initiated weekly FaceTime calls, so Dad and I could finally see each other weekly. He could have a virtual visitor. I wished we'd been able to do it since the beginning. During one phone call, Dad told me he was sad and depressed when I asked. I told him a couple of cheesy dad jokes.

"Why are frogs good at baseball?" I paused. "Because they know how to catch fly balls."

He at least halfway cracked a smile. I'd keep trying.

Jackie, Keith, and I sent him See's chocolate because he was open to that idea, again.

But still weeks later, the fact that Dad had suffered multiple strokes devastated me. Was there something we could've done to prevent it? Did they occur after I found him, or before? Is this why he was transported to the hospital from the homeless shelter?

Couldn't the universe cut my dad a break? He was a good guy. He'd been a great dad. He didn't deserve all of this. None of us did.

CHAPTER FIFTY-FOUR

THE RETURN

In the spring of 2021, our school returned to in-person learning. David had been able to return to attending class on campus at his middle school the previous semester.

Not that re-opening my high school helped—I didn't have more than a handful of students whose parents brought them back to campus. That meant my camera and microphone had to be constantly connected to Zoom and we teachers had to instruct online and in-person at the same time, responding to the questions from hands raised in class and questions posted in the text online. All of this while projecting slides with my lessons on the whiteboard and sharing my slides correctly through the Zoom screen sharing feature.

And that was all before noon. After lunch, we had to sit in our physical classrooms by ourselves with our cameras on in a usually empty Zoom virtual classroom to be available for students who had questions during the afternoon at-home asynchronous learning time. Meanwhile, we had to keep up with grading and continuing to modify instruction to provide digital resources for students. Basically, it was like taking everything we'd taught for nearly twenty years and modifying every single unit and creating digital versions of everything.

It was beyond exhausting.

On the bright side, because Leo and I couldn't rebook our wedding at the regional park, we instead landscaped our backyard, complete with paths, trees, and lighting, installed a gazebo, which Justin, Leo, and I put together, and prepared for a backyard wedding. Our friends and family were available, and, even better, Keith could walk me down my stone path aisle.

Three of my good friends—we had bonded during the Covid isolation—came with me to downtown LA to pick out fabric. I found a local tailor who helped me design and custom-fit the wedding dress of my dreams. Leo bought his tux, all of the boys had been fitted for suits, the DJ, photographer, videographer, photo booth, and barbecue caterer—slow cooked smoked brisket is the best!—had all been rebooked. Our wedding would be even better than I imagined. Dad would've loved the barbecue.

I eagerly counted down the days.

I also looked forward to my weekly FaceTime chats with Dad which I scheduled during my lunch at work. Because my friends and I opened each lesson with a joke-of-the-day, basically "dad jokes," I had an arsenal to sort through to share with Dad, all in the hopes of getting him to smile.

"Hey Dad, what about this one? I gave my handyman a to-do list, but he only did jobs one, three, and five. Know why?" Dad shook his head. "Turns out he only does odd jobs."

Dad either shrugged, nodded, blinked, or didn't react. Even if he wasn't laughing, the nursing assistants and CNAs cracked up at them, so at least I was amusing someone.

The CNA held up the phone to Dad, dressed in a hospital gown—apparently nobody insisted he get dressed every day. He was lying in bed.

"Would you like me and the boys to come out to see you in August?" I asked.

He gave me a slight nod, but his eyes maintained a blank stare.

By April, in-person visits at his nursing home resumed, so Dad had something to look forward to with Amy's visits. She also brought him clothes and anything else he needed.

"I was able to see your dad today," Amy said to me. "He was up in a Geri chair and they brought him down. Apparently, they get him up in this chair, because he insists that he can't walk and they need to help him, which

I know isn't true. I reminded him that he walked independently when we first met but today, he says that he didn't."

"I'm glad you're able to visit him again," I said. "I'm sure he's been lonely."

"Outwardly he appears the same, but he needs a shave. The first thing he said without prompting from me was, 'The mob is still after me.'"

I groaned. Not again. Would it ever go away? "That sucks Dad still has to deal with hallucinations and paranoia."

"It's pretty scary for him and he mentioned that he doesn't tell you because he needs to protect you. I don't know how reassuring that is but it certainly says a lot about how he feels about you."

"Yes, while it's nice to know he cares, it's upsetting he has these irrational fears now."

"Even though I've not known him to not be delusional, I recall you saying there were plenty of times that he was not and I'm sorry about this. The staff says that he does take his meds. I have a care plan meeting next week and I hope to discuss his case, too."

"I haven't gotten a chance to speak with him over the past two weeks, once because I missed the call, and the second week because I never got a call."

"I know he really enjoys your weekly video chats."

So, did I.

I came up with a plan to try to provide some familiar comfort for Dad. I asked Jackie to email me photos of her and her family, and I asked Keith the same. I bought a wallet filled with the clear pockets and filled each one with pictures of all of his children and grandchildren. I wanted him to enjoy life a little, too, so I told Ashley to make sure he had money in the wallet and encourage him to buy snacks, which I found out they offered to residents.

After Amy's next visit, I asked her if Dad needed anything.

"I didn't know," she said, "but I can ask. Last time I visited him, I bought him several shirts and pants. When I saw him today, he wasn't wearing any of them and the staff didn't know where they were."

"So, they lost them? I thought this place would be better about that."

"I assumed they'd label them. They always do that so things don't get lost although it's 'best laid plans.' In my experience sometimes things get lost anyway."

"If you bring him more clothes, would it be possible for you to label them? That's the only way he'll get them back after washing. I was thinking an obnoxious 'Joseph's' written across the backs in black sharpie might work."

She laughed. "Might help. I'd like to ask if he can get a haircut in their salon. I always recall him wearing it short. I suppose he may not care, but what do you think?"

"Yes, please." Then, remembering the last FaceTime call I had with him, I added: "Can you ask them to shave him, too?"

By the end of May, most of our world returned back to the new normal. Amy updated me after her visit with him on May 27.

"I visited with your dad this week. It was warm, so we met on the garden patio."

"He loves nature," I said, "so even if you can't drive him around the lake, I'm glad you got him outside."

"Me, too. Apparently, he's just had a phone call with Jackie. Overall, he doesn't change much to me and he looked good, dressed with his new shoes."

"At least his shoes didn't disappear."

"Yes, and on the positive side, he said he's sleeping better with the new pillow."

"Memory foam is better than the flat ones they have there. What's the downside?"

"He's still worried about his 'enemies.' He primarily shrugs his shoulders when I push him a little about the reality of this."

Was the medicine even working? I didn't have a degree in psychiatry, but I had hoped the drugs would've eased his suffering from schizophrenia. When would the world find a cure? But with only roughly one percent of the population suffering from it, would it ever be profitable for researchers to invest in discovering a cure?

Maybe one day, scientists would discover the genetic markers and find a way to reverse them, or shut off the ones that caused SMI. Maybe this didn't even make sense, but something had to eventually change. It would save so much money for all of society and so much heartache for the families and the individuals.

Just when I thought I was done with upsetting news, one afternoon, Justin, now twenty-four years old and living at home, approached me after we got into an argument over his finances. Rather than accumulating savings while he lived at home, he'd been accumulating debt. I tried to get him to understand how dangerous this habit would be for his future.

"Look at your credit card statement." I had highlighted all of the unnecessary expenses. "You're not saving money. We keep fighting about the same thing over and over again. It's a serious problem."

"Well, here's a solution," Justin said. "I'm moving out."

CHAPTER FIFTY-FIVE
Ohio

"What?" I shouted at Justin. "How are you going to move out if you don't have money?"

"I'll figure it out," he said.

Typical immature response. "Where?" Maybe he'd end up sleeping on a friend's couch.

"Dayton, Ohio."

"Ohio! Are you pissed off at me? What did I do for you to move across the country?"

"It's not that. I have a friend out there. He said it's cheap for me to get an apartment."

"How much is the rent? How are you going to pay for it?"

"Eight hundred a month for a big one-bedroom. I got offered a job."

Eight hundred? Okay, he had me there. Even a studio in Orange County cost around two thousand dollars. Still, Ohio was far from our family, far from me. "Doing what?"

"Building maintenance." He had earned his HVAC and EPA certifications through a local junior college.

"Is it a safe area?"

"Yes, don't worry."

"I'm your mom. Of course I'm going to worry. You decide to move clear across the country without any notice."

"Calm down. I'm not taking the job or moving until after the wedding and after you and Leo get back from your honeymoon. I'll move at the end of July. And by the way, it has nothing to do with our fight. I've been planning it for a while, but didn't say anything."

"Well, I appreciate you waiting until after the wedding. But, how do you know it's a good area? You've never even been to Ohio. Doesn't it snow?"

"I like the cold. And, let me put it this way, it's in a nice neighborhood, there's a Costco, a craft burger place, Cheesecake Factory and all the places there you like. My buddy knows the area. It's really nice. Plus, the complex has a lake they fully stock, so I could fish if I wanted to."

When I researched it online, his story checked out, and it was a manageable five-hour drive to Chicago. That meant that whenever I visited Justin, I'd be able to visit Dad.

"So, you're thinking of leaving at the end of July?" I asked. "You're just packing up your Civic and diving across the country by yourself?"

He nodded.

"No, you're not," I said. "I'll load up more stuff in the SUV and follow you there. I can cover the hotels and then we can do one final road trip together."

"You mean it? You're actually going to do that? That's a long drive."

"Of course I will. My baby's moving out."

So, we made plans. Together.

When I was Justin's age, my dad had already lost his mind and disappeared from our lives. If he'd been dead or a horrible dad, his absence would've been expected, but no one could have anticipated him leaving us all behind. I didn't want to leave Justin on his own.

I knew it wasn't Dad's fault, a SMI is not the person's fault, but I regretted his absence during all those years of my life. At least I could be there for Justin, in the way that I hoped my old dad would have been there for me.

CHAPTER FIFTY-SIX

The Trek

SUMMER 2021

My wedding was only ten days away. During her visits with Dad, Amy asked him if he'd be willing to record a special message for me, but the answer was always no. But that didn't prevent her from trying.

Leo's parents and sister flew in from New York and my mom was there—so all the parents, except Dad.

The weather was perfect while we snapped first look photos at the park alongside a lake and atop a wooden bridge. Leo serenaded me with Elton John's "Your Song," we exchanged rings and our self-written vows, ate, drank, and danced alongside our closest friends and family.

After our wedding, I sent Dad pictures of me in my soft white, A-line wedding dress with French bustles, and our rustic decorations, slices of wood with tin vases tied with burlap and purple ribbons, filled with purple and pink peonies. Amy shared the pics with Dad. I sent pics of me, Keith, and Jackie posing in the gazebo, the sheers lightly billowing in the breeze. I wanted these pictures to be added to the photos in his wallet.

And after I shipped Dad See's chocolate for his birthday in July, packed for my honeymoon, and prepared for Justin's move back East, I contacted Dad's nursing home to arrange a care meeting. Then on Friday, July 9, Leo and I departed LAX for the Dominican Republic for our honeymoon. I was glad that despite our hotel's Wi-Fi, our reception was spotty. That meant, at least until we landed back in LAX on Sunday, July 18, I could take a break from worries and have a chance to relax.

In late July, Justin and I packed up both his Civic and my SUV. I had no visibility with his things packed into the SUV like a Tetris puzzle from side to side and top to bottom, and I didn't trust my side mirrors alone. So, I needed Justin's help with lane changes. We stayed on the phone during most of the drive. I led the way, but whenever I needed to switch lanes, he'd took the lead by moving out first and holding a spot open for me so slide in, in front of him.

We traversed across 40-East through Flagstaff, Arizona; Amarillo, Texas; a private Corvette collection in a restored historical oil town in Texas; a brief venture in the Diamond Mine Park where we combed through the dirt only to leave, not with diamond, but with sunburns, thirst, and exhaustion; the best barbecue in Memphis, Tennessee; a ride on the Delta Riverboats at the Opryland Hotel in Nashville; and a tour deep inside Mammoth Caves in Kentucky. We arrived a week later in Dayton, Ohio where we delivered his belongings, went bargain shopping for used furniture, and stocked up his new apartment.

I reconfirmed the details of Dad's care meeting and visit—Amy would meet us there—then picked up David from the easily-accessible Dayton Airport.

On Sunday, August 1, David and I made the trek to Chicago to visit Dad. First thing on the agenda? Chili cheese dogs and a cake shake at Portillo's and picking up more Fannie May chocolates and Mint Meltaways for Dad.

The next morning, we drove up to the new facility. Even from the outside, with its charming brick construction and close proximity to the lake, I already liked it better than the old place. The interior hallways didn't have peeling footboards nor were we greeted with a putrid stench like the old place. The staff members, especially Fred, middle-aged with a thin build and well-accentuated smile lines, and Ashley, thirty-something with a full head of blonde curls and big brown eyes, were warm and welcoming.

David and I exited the elevator and entered Dad's room and each gave him a mostly one-sided hug. At least he was dressed for the day. While David said hello, I pulled open Dad's nightstand and cabinets drawers. It was empty except for two recent birthday cards from me and Jackie. His wallet wasn't there. I swore he had more clothing than I found hanging in his closet. Even the teddy bear Justin and I had gotten him at the previous facility was not there. Not again. I took a mental note to bring that up later with the staff.

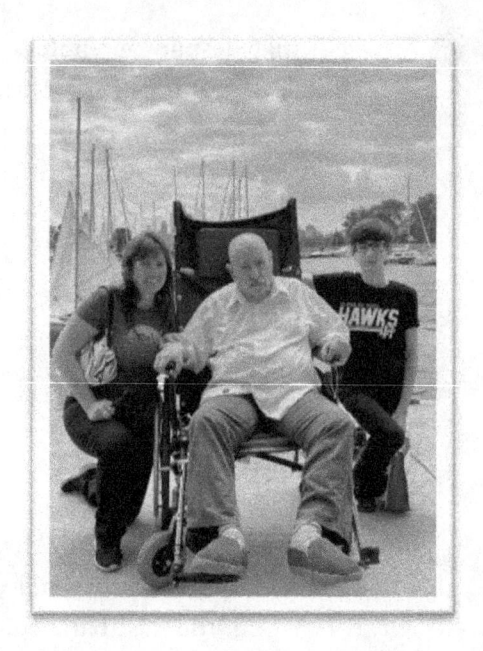

The nursing assistants eased Dad into a wheelchair-like chair, which more closely resembled a hospital-style blue-green recliner on wheels. I turned around at hearing a familiar voice, one of empathy and calm. Although I'd seen Amy over FaceTime, greeting her in person filled me with joy. Even with a mask on, her eyes showcased her smile.

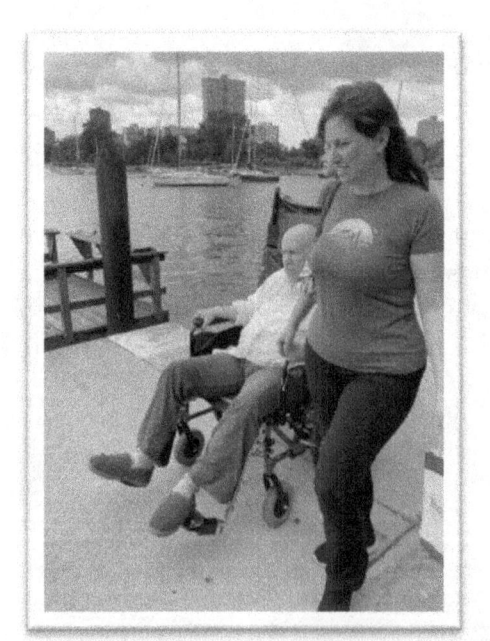

She and I realized Dad's Merrell shoes were missing. We exchanged a glance. She shook her head and helped him into a pair of old slippers and wheeled him down the elevator and outdoors.

"I thought it might be nice to walk across the street," she said.

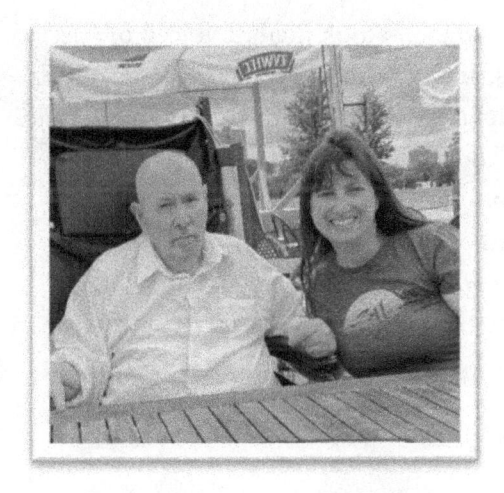

"It's not far and we'll pass by the docks. There's a hot dog stand at the end but we can always go somewhere else if you prefer."

We were a sight: Amy pushing Dad in a reclined hospital chair, with David and I following alongside.

"Look at the boats, Dad." I pointed to the rows of boats with their sails furled. "It's a gorgeous day."

He was heavy on the nods and shrugs, but, like usual, light on words. I wiped mustard off the corner of his mouth so we could take pictures.

I tried hard while we were seated on the outdoor dining patio, as the photos later showed, to act silly enough to get a tiny smile out of Dad. Although I wasn't successful—he appeared lost inward, deep in thought—he did squint through the sunshine and glance out at Lake Michigan. That was good enough.

Back at the nursing home, Amy accompanied us out back to the garden where Dad's care team was assembling.

Each person gave me an update: Yes, he's getting occupational therapy; Other than a couple times they got him out for an activity where he proceeded to sit in the back in a wheelchair rather than participate, he wasn't doing activities. We realized a barrier to getting him out more was that assistants needed to get Dad dressed and ready to go, or he was missing opportunities to be persuaded to go more often. This basic detail and lack of coordination surprised me, but a plan was put in place to address it.

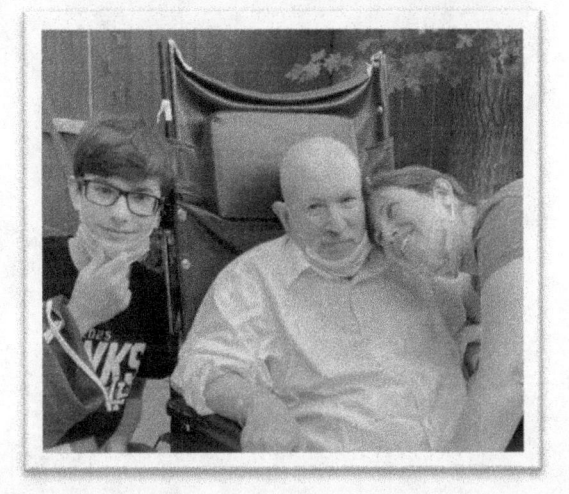

Dad's psych meds were stable, when he took them. I voiced my desire to continue weekly FaceTime calls, and we handled other business details.

But it wasn't until everyone, including Amy, said goodbyes and left me, Dad, and David to visit, that Dad motioned me closer. David sat back out of earshot, playing games on his phone.

When I was close enough, Dad opened his mouth to finally speak.

I leaned forward to better hear him.

Dad whispered, "I was molested."

CHAPTER FIFTY-SEVEN

Accusations

"That's why they moved me," Dad said. "The guy in my last room molested me and touched me in the privates. He grabbed me."

I wasn't sure whether this memory was true or not. "Did it happen more than once?"

He nodded. "I punched him in the shoulder and put cold water on him. And I wasn't the first one. That asshole did something to someone else so they put him in a room by himself."

My jaw dropped open and I flagged over a staff member and demanded to speak to the administration regarding Dad's accusation. Why in hell didn't someone notify me? I knew they had recently relocated Dad, but no one had told me why. Clearly, this was something worth notifying a family member about.

While we waited, Dad elaborated on other complaints.

Three administrators came outside, with solemn expressions, with business cards in hand and forms, a notebook, and pen.

"I can assure you," the Director said. "If we had known anything about this, we would've called you."

"Sexual abuse is infuriating. The fact I wasn't immediately notified is absolutely unacceptable."

"We agree. That behavior is not tolerated here. Now, Joseph, if you wouldn't mind sharing the details with us, we need to investigate and file a police report. Then, pending the outcome, we may need to remove this other man from our facility."

"First of all," I said. "Before we get into the details, I want another complaint noted: why is he always in a hospital gown? I see that during my weekly Facetime calls. And after he fell, which thank goodness the staff phoned to inform me of, why doesn't anybody help him get out of bed? He's bedridden. When he gets frustrated and gets up on his own, that's when he falls. Nurses need to get him up and in the chair throughout the day."

They nodded and took notes with the distinct demeanor and facial expressions I'd expect from representatives who feared a lawsuit was coming.

"And another thing," I continued. "Why are all of his things missing? His pillow, his clothes, his teddy bear, even his brand-new shoes! And the most important thing—his wallet full of family photos, the only photos he has."

They scribbled more notes.

It was late by the time David and I returned to our hotel, the one where Justin worked, in Dayton. I returned a missed call from the nursing home administrator.

"We made a police report, a report to the state, and a report with our corporate office. I've interviewed our staff. They knew there was a problem between Joseph and this other man, but we didn't realize this is what it was. There were only the two of them in that room from June 29 until July 12. After hearing shouting, when staff entered the room, they caught this other man holding on to your father's leg. Thinking they were just arguing, we moved Joseph."

"Honestly, I'm shocked and beyond disappointed that no one told me. I only found out he moved rooms when my sister told me. I can never get a hold of Dad when I call."

"We're recommending psychotherapy for your dad, and we'll see how that goes. You have my word that I will personally be in contact with you every couple of days to update you."

"I want a copy of the police report."

"Absolutely. Not a problem." She paused. "When the police asked Joseph why he didn't tell anyone sooner, he pointed to me and Ashley and said, 'Well, I'm telling them now.'"

"I doubt you heard what Dad told me yesterday when I asked him why he didn't report it sooner, he said, 'the guy said he'd punch me and I was scared,' so he was too intimidated to tell."

"That's useful information. Thank you. I'll add that into the reports. We examined your dad today and didn't find any signs of abuse."

"Why would you find anything if he hasn't been around Dad in nearly three weeks?"

Within days, a police officer called to interview me as they continued the investigation.

A week and a half later, after David and I had completed our cross-country drive back to California, Ashley called. "With all of the moves, we're sorry your dad's things were misplaced. I wanted to let you know we did find your dad's wallet with the pictures, his clothes, and his shoes, basically all of his belongings… except the bear. To be honest, we're not even sure if it came over from his other old facility."

"Good. And how is he doing?"

"He's been getting up and dressed and chatting more with the Activities Director."

Well, now isn't that amazing? I rolled my eyes. Not a coincidence that this changed after I spoke directly to the Facility Director. And if this could happen to us, with Amy's help and all of our resources, and me with all of my experience and knowledge gained through my ten years on the Board of Directors NAMI-OC, then how on Earth were other families navigating the mental health and nursing home systems?

"Do you think the abuse really happened?" Jackie asked. "It's horrible."

"Or if it was as bad as he described?" Keith asked. "Because if so, there needs to be some consequences for the facility to cover up something like that."

"Honestly," I said, "there's no way to know for sure. Obviously, this other guy is a problem if he grabbed Dad's leg, but whether or not anything sexually happened? No one can prove anything. It's equally possible that Dad's mind exaggerated it, that he hallucinated, or, maybe that it is true. A lot of things he has told us in the past, like the devil possessing Hilda and seeing a man with a snake's tongue, clearly weren't true."

Either way, we couldn't prove anything. The police and administrators investigated. They interviewed patients and staff. No one else had made any similar accusations about the patient in question. There was no evidence. So, we couldn't dwell on it. Just prevent it going forward, and move on.

When a loved one has hallucinations and delusions from a SMI, family is often left wondering what's reality and what's not.

CHAPTER FIFTY-EIGHT

THE PSYCH WARD

A FEW WEEKS after my visit to Chicago, Dad was transferred to a psych hospital for suicidal ideation. I wondered if his increased depression was because of the alleged abuse, or because he felt lonely after David and I left. Perhaps it was a bit of both.

After he was released back to his facility, I stayed in regular contact with Ashley, the Director of the Facility, the Director of Nursing and other staff, oftentimes with Amy's help.

We sent constant emails back and forth.

Wednesday, September 1, 2021
Amy, 12:53 PM: I visited with your dad today and we talked about him seeing the dentist. Can we also get an OT evaluation for Joseph's left hand? It appears more contracted and I wonder if he could use a brace. Also, he's feeling much more depressed lately and has some passive suicidal ideation (related to his mob enemies). Denies voices telling him to do anything but he thinks they can get in his room and hurt him. Can the doctor see him please? It couldn't hurt. Let me know what you think.

Amanda, 2:12 PM: Yes, please keep me updated on this (dental care and OT). It sounds like his psych medicines need to be changed. If the delusions are present and causing him distress, isn't there something the psychiatrist can do? Who is the current psychiatrist seeing my dad?

Amy, 2:16 PM: Looks like they have to send Joseph out to ED for psych eval due to his suicidal ideation. I'm not sure if the hospital will talk to me without your permission but I will try. I forgot to add that he is again refusing medications on and off. This sure doesn't help, darn.

Amanda, 2:36 PM: Again? He needs to see a psychiatrist to adjust his medication. I feel like the hospitals just make changes to his medicine without the follow up. What about the injection? I think that lasts for three months. They also have a schizophrenia medication that is dissolvable. What about that one?

Amy, 3:27 PM: I agree. The injections last a month but I think they're hesitant because of his age. The olanzapine may already be the dissolvable one, I'll ask.

While I'd been communicating with Amy, Ashley left me a voicemail asking me to call back. She confirmed Dad had been transferred to Thorek Hospital for a psych eval.

Amy, Friday, Sept. 3, 2021, 7:35 AM: Today I called to check on Joseph and he'd been transferred to the medical unit for a low heart rate (40s to 50s). I think it was precautionary and it could very well be in the normal range for him but I'm not sure. He's been refusing meds there and after he's seen they'll send him back down to the psych unit. I'll push again for long acting [injections] but I'm not sure they'll do it (he may need cardiac clearance) or do it against his will. It doesn't make sense but hospitals interpret POAs differently.

Amy, Thursday, Sept. 9, 3:01 PM: Joseph was transferred back to behavioral health. The nurse said he is taking his meds; I suspect they have the skills to reassure him.

Amanda, 6:42 PM: Glad to hear he's taking medicine. Yesterday when I talked to the social worker, he told me Dad still hadn't been taking his medicine. I told them I wanted them to try to stabilize him on medicine before sending him back to the nursing home again.

Amy, Sunday, September 12, 12:32 PM: So relieved to hear Joseph is getting a long-acting injection!! Thank goodness. Staff has been very nice and very patient. I think he may be there a few more days but he's in no hurry… he likes it.

Amanda, Thursday, September 16, 3:11 PM: I asked them to call you but I'm not sure if they did. Two days ago, I was notified that my dad was already back in the nursing home. The man from the nursing home who phoned me said Dad seemed the same, still worried about the mafia. We are hoping that over the next week or two when the medicine kicks in, the delusions will subside. I guess they need to give him a shot every 2 to 3 weeks according to the nurse who spoke with me from Thorek earlier. When do you think you'll be able to visit with him?

Amy, 3:21 PM: I was there the day he got back; they told me although I didn't get to see him. I'll go next week. My expectation will be that he will be less paranoid and more consistent with taking his meds. I'm not sure that fixed delusion will go away completely but hope that it is less intense and that he will feel safer and more at peace. The dose was on the low side maybe because of his age. I give the injections a lot at work but my patients are younger. Our goal is often to keep people functional, out of the hospital and safe. I'll reach out to the nurse practitioner who works with him at the nursing home and at the hospital after I see him… By the way I've been reading your book

Amanda, Saturday, September 18, 3:21 PM: I wish Dad could have a happier last few years of his life. I would hate to be living through the delusions and paranoia that he is experiencing. Is there any way if you can bring him Big Macs from McDonald's when you visit him? I'll send you money for them. I hope you enjoy the book if enjoy is the right word for it…or find it interesting/helpful.

Amy, 5:29 PM: I'm happy to bring him McDonald's. I'm only about a third of the way through, oh Amanda, what a long road it's been for all of you. He's so lucky to have you.

From the Psychotherapist to Amanda, Monday, September 20, 3:36 PM: I wanted to reach out to provide a quick update on your father. I met with him today for our weekly therapy session, and he seemed significantly less symptomatic. He informed me that he is no longer afraid of his "enemies" and currently feels safe/comfortable in the building. He also reported a reduction in depressive symptoms (i.e. no longer experiencing "heavy depression" like he was before). Although he continues to present with delusional thinking and depression/anxiety, it seems that the new medication might be working.

Joseph also mentioned you during our session. He wanted me to let you know that he'd like to speak to you whenever you are available. I'm hoping that this new medication continues to reduce the severity of his symptoms - I will keep you updated!

Amanda to Amy, 4:28 PM: It sounds like hopefully the injection is helping. I hope they keep up with the injections. I did phone my dad and talked to him briefly, but he couldn't seem to hear me very well so it wasn't a very fruitful conversation. At least he knows I called.

Amy, Tuesday, September 22, 4:22 PM: I visited with your dad today. I brought a Big Mac which he loved and we watched your video. He appeared more internally preoccupied then last time I saw him but he was able to acknowledge and discuss it which is actually good (it's always about his enemies). I haven't heard back from Ashley, but he told me he's taking his meds …. I need to verify that with her of course. I always tell him it is my goal to help him quiet those voices and reassure him that he is safe and not suffering with fear. I often feel like I'm not giving you the best news but I do think that's a realistic hope. These delusions are so chronic that I don't think they will ever be gone completely. I think if he goes to activities and is up that he has the chance to be distracted from them.

We need to get an order for OT eval for a brace of some kind for his left hand. It's possible he won't allow or wear one but it's worth the effort. It seems like those 3 fingers are stiffer. This is from those little strokes we talked about. He has good range of motion with his thumb and index finger.

Amanda, 6:50 PM: I'm glad he enjoyed your visit and the Big Mac. Yesterday, his therapist told me that Dad mentioned me during their session and wanted to talk with me. I phoned him last night but it was difficult for him to hear me so it wasn't a productive conversation.

Things continued in this manner. Our goal was the same as always: to make Dad as comfortable as possible, to quiet the voices and calm his fears, which would hopefully keep at the nursing home and out of the psych wards.

Now that Justin was in Ohio, I couldn't bear the thought of him spending the holidays out there all by himself. He tried to convince me that the kitten he just adopted would keep him company.

"Can't you come home for Christmas?" I asked.

"No, Mom," he said. "I'm the new guy and don't have the days to take off."

"Fine. Then we'll fly out to you."

I booked flights for Leo, David, and me to visit Dad—and finally introduce my husband to my dad—then Justin from December 21 through December 28.

To prepare for our visit with Dad, I asked Amy to buy him a set of checkers and chess. Otherwise, without a planned activity, I imagined we'd spend hours staring at each other in silence.

Because that's pretty much what I felt my phone and video conversations had become—one-sided, me and the wall.

CHAPTER FIFTY-NINE

CHECKERS AND CHESS

TUESDAY, DECEMBER 21, 2021

To lighten the mood, as soon as we got to the nursing home, I put in an order for Carson's ribs, coleslaw, potatoes, and cornbread. It was dark and cold outside, so the four of us sat, Leo, David, and I in plastic chairs, and Dad in his wheelchair in an empty dining room waiting for the food.

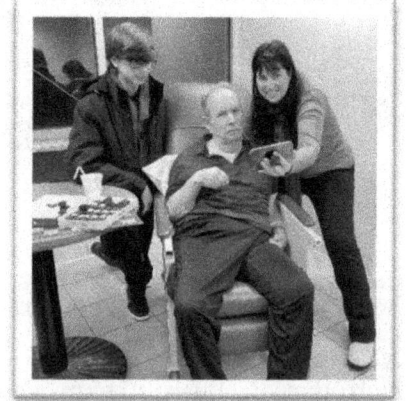

My phone buzzed. "It's here." I motioned to Leo and David. "Talk while I go to pay."

I came back in, with a security guard's help, carrying bags full of food. When the door opened, the scene wasn't what I'd hoped for. Leo sat on one end, checking the email on his phone, David sat on another end, playing games on his phone, and Dad sat in the center staring off into space.

While we ate, I tried my best. "Dad, Leo here works in computers like you did."

Dad nodded.

"Leo, want to tell Dad what you do?"

Leo started to give a brief explanation but Dad interrupted him. "Not the same."

"Yes, you worked on mainframe computers, right, Dad?"

He nodded.

"Hey, David, can you tell Grandpa about school?"

"It's going alright," David said then glared at me and shrugged.

I sighed and finished my meal.

I had better luck after we relocated to the library where David and I took turns playing checkers and chess with Dad.

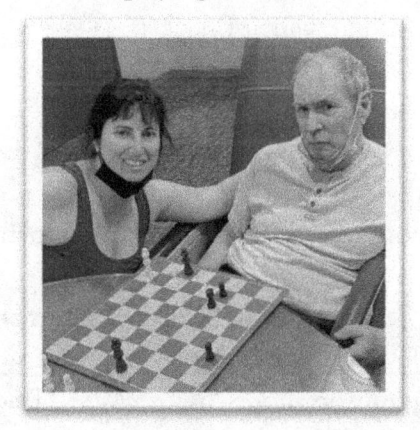

I remembered being a little younger than David when Dad taught me to play chess. After a few moves of our pawns, bishops, knights, and the occasional castling, I'd inadvertently make a dumb move that endangered my queen or king.

Rather than destroy me, Dad said, "Mmm… are you sure you want to do that?"

"Well, I thought so, until you said that." I returned my bishop and stared at the board. "Why? What?" Then I saw it. His knight would have taken out my bishop. "Oh." So, I slid my queen across the board instead, in striking distance of his king. "Check."

"Mmm… is that what you want to do?"

"Yes? No?" Then I saw one of his lowly pawns could easily capture my queen. I slid her back and moved a pawn instead to capture one of his.

He nodded. This is not to say that Dad let me win, even as a kid. On the contrary, I never beat him, instead only managing to tie him a handful of times.

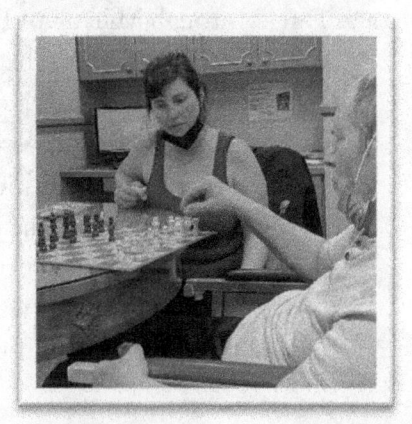

David, on the other hand, had a chess mind like Dad's without the consequences I faced with my impatience. But when he played his grandpa, while I helped Dad remember how the pieces moved, I noticed David purposely not playing his best game. When there were only a few pieces left on the board, David and his grandpa split the wins.

At Checkers, David who could destroy many opponents—he reminded me a lot of Dad—played cautiously, at times deliberating opening himself up to attack. In the end, Dad won, but he didn't acknowledge it with anything more than a nod.

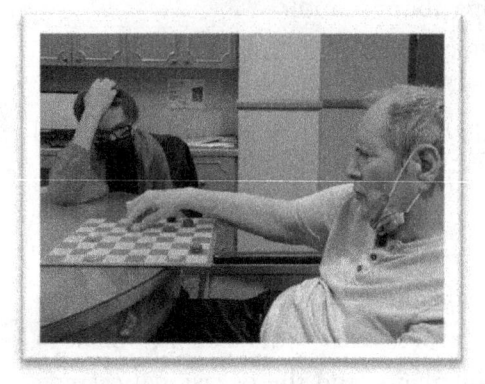

"That was nice of you," I said to David as we were leaving. "You let him win at Checkers."

David laughed. "Not really. I mean initially, yes. But in the end, I made an honest mistake and he beat me fair and square."

How lucky was I to have such a thoughtful caring son? Two of them in fact.

We hopped on the Lake Shore Expressway bus and while we returned to our hotel, I daydreamed about all the years that weren't, years of Dad playing checkers and chess with his grandson, hours of *Scrabble*... Dad teaching his grandson how to play poker and how to bet in blackjack. Late night movies and hot fudge sundaes, museums on the weekend, the occasional Greek festival.

But, alas, those weren't the cards life had dealt us.

It was so cold the next day—barely hitting double digits—that I wore a facemask while walking just to keep my nose, lips, and chin from freezing. I led Leo and David through Millenium Park.

We did an escape room that took place in a fake jail cell. We wasted so much time trying to escape in the dark with a dim flashlight not realizing until near the end that we could've turned on the light switch the entire time, but we hadn't tried. Why is it that sometimes the easy things are right in front of us, but we can't find them?

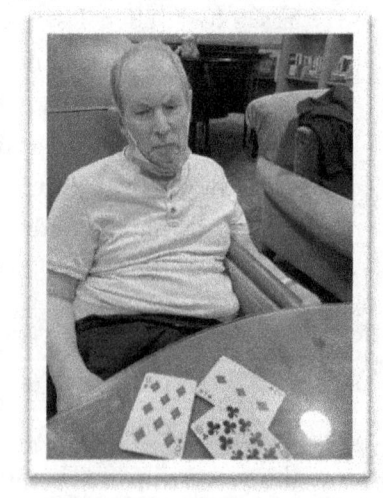

If only life were so simple. If only there was a light switch that I could flip to clearly illuminate everything, especially Dad's SMI, making it all much easier to deal with.

My favorite stop, much like my dad's, was The Field Museum. This time, I wasn't preoccupied like I had been during our last visit. Without having to worry about POA docs, I was able to enjoy the dioramas of animals in their natural habitats, the dinosaur exhibits, and the gems.

At the end of our day, David stopped in the gift shop. "Can we get grandpa something?" He held out a brown stuffed animal. "He said he liked bears and he lost the other one. This one even is wearing a shirt that says Chicago."

"That's the state flag." I smiled. Maybe a stuffed animal would keep him company.

On our next visit to see Dad, along with a box of chocolates, David brought the bear.

"Grandpa." He held it out. "We got this for you because I know you like bears. It has a Chicago shirt on it." He handed it to Dad who gripped it in his good hand, not the one that remained clutched, presumably from a stroke.

Then David reached over and gave his grandpa a hug. I looked away to keep from crying.

CHAPTER SIXTY

THE SPEECH THERAPIST

FEBRUARY 8, 2022, 1:11 PM

I missed a call from Chicago. When I checked my voicemail, I expected to hear the usual, "Hi, this is so-and-so at the facility. Please give us a call back." But the one I received that day was not like the others:

> Hi, Amanda, I'm the Speech Therapist at the facility and I'm calling regarding your dad, Joseph. I heard you have some questions about his diet. I did pick him up for swallowing because the nurse told me he was coughing while he was eating. And I did a video swallow study on him just to kind of see what was going on because we had an inconsistent cough when he would eat and I was wondering if he was possibly aspirating.
>
> And I found out that he was having some issues with liquids, thin liquids, and nectar thick liquids. There was some aspiration going on. So, they recommended that I put him on honey-thick liquids. He wasn't aspirating or anything with that but I still have him on my caseload, just monitoring him to see him, making sure he's okay with his current diet. He's on a mechanical soft diet. That's soft cooked solid food and the meat is ground up so it's easier for

him to chew. So, if you have any questions for me, please give me a call, if you want to talk some more about his diet.

Aspirating with eating? I had never heard of such a thing. I soon learned the term dysphagia and that it could be caused by, among other things, strokes or dementia.

I called them back for more information. Although the speech therapist wasn't available, I did get a hold of a nurse and we had a difficult discussion.

"You know," she said. "This is common with dementia patients."

"I didn't know he had dementia." I'd never gotten solid medical confirmation that he had Alzheimer's either but knew they were similar. "What do we do? Can the speech therapist work with him to cure it?"

"It doesn't work like that. We see that here, as patients get older. We change their diet to thickened liquids, softer food."

"She mentioned the word aspirate. What does that mean?"

"If we're not careful, and he aspirates, that means food gets into his lungs and he could get pneumonia, so we want to prevent that."

"Will it get worse?"

"Usually. It's something we recommend the families talk about when it gets worse. Eventually they can't eat and they need a feeding tube or—"

"Dad does not want a feeding tube."

"Don't worry. It's not an issue now. But we noticed the coughing, which is why we had him evaluated."

Which I was glad they had. But I had never heard of dysphagia before. I wondered: when did Dad have the strokes, what caused them, and did they lead to this swallowing issue? Or did Dad have Alzheimer's like we feared and that led to this?

Either way, the result was the same. At least for now though, the honey-thick liquids and mechanically softened foods were working.

Still, the fact that Dad was having trouble swallowing wasn't a good sign.

CHAPTER SIXTY-ONE

Misunderstood

APRIL 2022

How could we celebrate Jackie's fiftieth birthday with Keith and I down in Southern California while she was up there?

"I can't take time off work," Keith said.

"I can head up during my Spring Break," I said. "I was thinking of surprising her with a weekend stay at a local hotel, maybe some wine tasting."

"It might be nice to take her to the spa to get a massage."

"And a pedicure and manicure?"

"Just tell me how much. Since you're paying for the hotel and food, I'll cover the other costs. I'm glad she'll have at least one of us up there."

After my plane touched down in their tiny airport, I met Jackie right outside and we held each other in a long hug. No matter whether or not we argued at times, she was my sister and we both loved each other.

We talked over each other trying to catch up with everything that had transpired in our lives since we last saw each other. Usually, we'd try to get together for Christmas, but because Leo, David, and I flew out to Ohio to be with Justin, we didn't get to see each other.

Jackie and I couldn't leave for the hotel though until I had a chance to visit with my brother-in-law Jim and my nieces and get in some revered game time—dominoes, *Splendor*, *Scrabble*. Then Jackie and I were off on our mini-vacation.

"Bring your swimsuit," I reminded her. A hot tub sounded great to both of us.

We celebrated her birthday the entire weekend: Wine tasting at the winery on a vineyard, a movie at the theater, the warmth of the hot tub, delicious food, and more.

While I enjoyed her company, there was a dark undertone to my mood, which I hadn't even realized until she pointed it out over lunch one day.

"Are you okay?" Jackie, attuned as ever, picked up the subtleties.

"Yeah, why?" I sipped my drink.

"Something's off with you… I can't quite place my finger on it. But you seem different… more… apathetic."

"How so?"

"Whenever we talk about Dad, even mental illness in general, you're not the same. Are you still on the Board of Directors?"

"Yeah, but I think I'm going to retire from the board this summer. It'll have been ten years. And, honestly, I'm just tired. I'm tired of dealing with everything. Difficult students at school, mental health crises, discussing mental health at conferences, talking to people about mental illness because of my book, dealing with Dad, and all that crap."

"You spend a lot of time taking care of things with Dad. I know Keith and I appreciate everything you do. You know that, right?"

"Does someone else want to take over? I'm just mentally done."

She eyed me for a moment. "What changed? You've changed."

"I searched for him for ten years. Then we found him and you know the conversations are very one-sided, I don't even know how you keep him on the phone for so long, but it's always something. The doctors, the bills, getting calls that he's screaming at the staff, his medicine is off, he's not taking his medicine, the mob is after him… I just can't… I can't do it anymore."

"I've been noticing the difference in you," she said. "You used to… I don't know… care more."

I stared at her blankly and took another sip of my drink, stuffed a French fry in my mouth and shrugged. She was right. I used to care more.

I don't know when things had changed, but they had. I hadn't realized it until that moment.

I sighed. "Now I know how Hilda felt."

"Well," Jackie said, bitterly. "We wouldn't know because she's cut herself off from the family."

"I don't think it's as simple as that. If you were in her shoes, how would you feel?"

"About us? Or about Dad?"

"Everything's connected."

She stared at me then a realization came over her and she nodded. "It's too much."

Family member caregivers can only take so much stress in taking care of a loved one with an SMI before the intrinsic rewards run dry and it becomes work and the work becomes a burden, which means your loved one becomes a burden. Then comes the guilt, but the guilt can't change the reality, especially when it usually falls on the shoulders of one person—the mom, a spouse, a sibling, and in our case, the middle child. While everyone else gets to carry on with their lives, the caregiver becomes an identity unto itself. A selfless, thankless one.

I thought back to the last couple years—talking to attorneys while shopping for my wedding dress, listening to Dad's crazy talk, him proselytizing to me the day before my wedding, contacting Dad's caregivers before the ink was dry on my marriage certificate at the courthouse, handling his medical care on my lunch breaks at work, researching and sending emails before and after dinner, checking my email first thing in the morning for news on Dad, rushing to answer the phone whenever a Chicago number showed up.

This was what my life had become—intertwined with his.

And, selfish or not, I wanted my life back.

We ate a few more minutes in silence, but Jackie kept glancing up at me. I sank my teeth into my burger and tried to forget about Dad.

"Are you getting compensated for being Dad's POA?" Jackie asked.

"No." I looked up at her. "Why would I be?"

"I just assumed you were. I know a lot of people do."

"No, I've never taken any money for anything. He's our dad."

"Well," she said. "Maybe you should."

And like that, Jackie set the wheels in motion, and she and Keith decided something needed to change and that I needed to be compensated for taking care of Dad.

I've never been motivated by money; otherwise, I wouldn't be teaching. I would've stayed in finance. Still, there's something to be said for getting something back for all of the effort expended. I felt more appreciated. It reawakened my ability to want to do more.

I realized there was a different path for everyone. I understood Jackie's decision to be on the sidelines, and for Hilda to step back, and for Keith to completely cut himself off. I didn't blame them, but I had to do more. I couldn't give up on Dad. It wasn't in me. Just like they couldn't control who they were and what they needed, this was who I was and what I needed to do.

I had Jackie and Keith to thank for that, which inadvertently trickled down to me being able to do more to help Dad. If Jackie hadn't picked up on my feelings, even though I didn't recognize them, and if Keith hadn't agreed and pushed for what he felt was fair, too, I soon may have lost the ability to care.

Apathy is dangerous, not just for the caretaker, but for the patient, too.

Before the dinner plates were cleared, I flagged over our server.

"It's my sister's birthday," I said. "Do you have anything with chocolate that you can put a candle in?"

After Jackie made a wish, we dug in to the rich, chocolate layered cake.

Jackie licked the frosting off her fork.

"By the way," she said. "Do you remember the disagreement we had last time we visited Dad in Chicago, after his heart attack?"

"Disagreement? You mean fight?" How could I forget?

"It was hurtful how you snapped at me instead of being kind and understanding when I was upset."

I didn't want to rehash old grievances. "Yeah. I know it sounds mean, but we didn't have time for your tears. We only had a very limited window of time to talk to the people we had to and we barely made it there as it was."

"Oh, I didn't realize that." She paused. "You know why I was crying?"

"Something about your mom and grandma and brothers plus Dad."

"Yeah, but you don't know what led up to that moment."

"Go on…"

She relayed how her doctor had changed her medicine right before the trip and she hadn't slept at all for two nights in a row. But that wasn't what threw her over the edge.

While I was fast asleep, comfy and cozy in the guest room, and her brother had already left for an early morning shift at work, she took a nice warm shower to relax enough to hopefully be able to get some sleep.

As soon as she lathered shampoo into her hair, the water turned from hot to freezing cold, and not California cold, but middle-of-the-winter, pipes might freeze, below freezing cold.

She screamed and jumped out of the water stream and tried to adjust the temperature. Her skin stung from contact with the water. Nothing worked. Turned it off and on again. Nope.

Dripping wet, with suds dripping down her shoulders, she hobbled her way over to the sink, leaned her head over it, and turned on the hot water. What came out was liquid ice. She screamed again and jumped back. And due to the fact that her brother kept his thermostat on the low end, her skin prickled with goosebumps.

She wrapped a towel—small enough to be a hand towel, and a robe, and another towel, and streaked from the hallway bathroom to her brother's bathroom shower. She twisted the hot water knob, but the results were the same.

Beyond tired and frustrated, she turned on his sink, bowed her head over the sink and did her best to get the soap off while her hands reddened and stung from the cold. It was after that, that she got dressed, sat on his bedroom carpet, stared at family photos on the wall, and cried for lost time.

"So, you were running around the house naked with shampoo dripping from your hair?"

She nodded. "And remember I hadn't slept in two days."

"Damn, that's funny," I said. "And I slept through the whole thing. Did I tell you how warm the shower was that I took before bed that night?"

She scowled and lightly punched me in the shoulder.

"Okay, I forgive you," I said with a grin. "Because after all, you are my favorite sister."

"Your only sister." She rolled her eyes, but we were good after that.

Often the assumptions we make about each other are wrong.

CHAPTER SIXTY-TWO

"Are You There, Dad?"

SUMMER 2022

For Dad's birthday I once again sent a box of See's along with the message: Happy Birthday, Dad! I hope these chocolates bring you some joy. Love, Amanda

Although I hadn't been communicating frequently with Melody about anything other than Dad's finances, I was surprised to get her email: "I just wanted to let you know I'm leaving in a couple weeks. Kevin will be taking over on this account as the Trust Officer. Alanna, another member on our team, will assist as the Trust Administrator for your dad's account."

I sent her a reply, "Thank you so much for letting me know. And thank you for everything you've done for my dad over the years, including helping me find him. I appreciate you so much, and without us working together, it's quite possible my dad might not be here today! So, as you move on, I just want you to know you made such a difference in our lives. If you ever want to keep in touch, you know my email address."

Candace had left the month before, shortly after another company acquired theirs.

I tried not to read too much into it, but it felt like a red flag.

It also meant that I had to retell Dad's story to our new team, Kevin and Alanna.

The frustrating thing was trying to get Dad to go to activities—he still had an issue with his clasped-shut left hand. He didn't want to wear the wrist brace because it hurt, but not wearing the brace was making his hand worse. They said some of this was likely from the strokes.

Jackie tried to FaceTime him but she found out, as I knew, it's frustrating because it's a one-sided conversation. Even with Amy prodding Dad to answer Jackie's questions, it was mostly the same.

The staff tried to help, but they had a lot to do and couldn't sit there for half an hour holding the phone for him. I gave up trying to call. It would just end up with Dad repeating, "I can't hear you" and me repeating, "Are you there Dad?" and all this after thirty minutes of trying to get him on the phone, which mostly resulted with me hanging up in irritation. It just felt useless.

The nurse practitioner updated me, "Sometimes Joseph acts helpless. He tries to get others to feed him. It's hard to tell how much is ability versus willingness or lack of motivation."

"Is he taking his meds?" I asked. "Because when I can actually talk to him, he's distracted. I can see it in his eyes. He indicated to Amy that it's the voices again."

"He is, according to the staff."

"Maybe he can't hear me? And his fingers are clenched. And he can't walk."

"The strokes affected his mobility."

"And dementia affects the ability to swallow." How it did was above my level of medical knowledge and I probably wouldn't understand the terms if she told me. "At his last place, he used to get a lot of UTIs."

"Here, we continue to check his hydration levels."

He did seem to be getting better medical care there.

I filled Jackie in on the details. "I don't know much about dementia," I said, "but I think they put that on grandma's death certificate. The swallow issue? It's hard to keep up with everything. It's just so frustrating."

"I don't want to get like this when I'm older," Jackie said. "I have enough aches and pains already."

"The only things that bring Dad joy are the Big Mac, fries, and Cokes Amy brings him."

"That's still the same." She laughed. "Some things, like chocolate, barbecue ribs, and big Macs, never change."

While I could no longer track Justin's finances, I knew he was working full time, paying his rent every month, and keeping his cat well cared for.

I missed him. I had to find an excuse to see him soon, but traveling around Christmas was such a nightmare. At least I had a four-day weekend in November. And better yet? The Eagles were playing a Veterans benefit concert in Columbus, Ohio.

"I'm heading back East to see my son in November," I said to Amy.

"So, you'll be stopping by here?" she asked. "Do you want to set up another care team meeting?"

"Yes. I'll be in Chicago on November tenth." Thinking of the new people at the trust company whom I didn't have the same emotional connection to, I added, "I also set up a meeting with Kevin and Alanna."

"Well, I'm sure your dad will be glad to see you." She paused. "He's had a long-acting injection ordered, but he's been refusing it. The NP is going to try to encourage him to accept it, but, again, they can't legally force it."

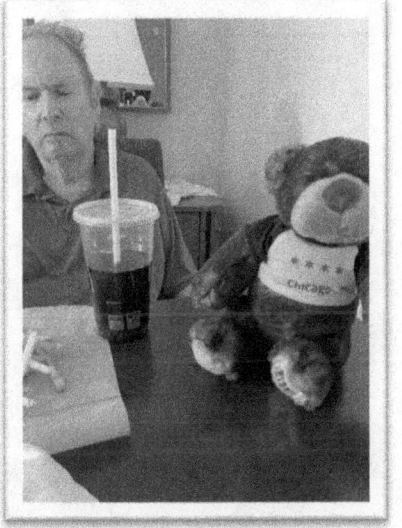

"If he keeps refusing, he's definitely going to get worse. I don't know what will happen from there. Maybe he refuses food, maybe he gets belligerent. If he has erratic behavior, is angry and mean, will they kick him out of the facility? If so, where would he go?"

"Please don't worry, they have far worse residents and they manage behaviors like this often. I'd be very surprised if that would ever happen. We can always problem solve."

It was reassuring to have someone in my corner, someone to help me work through the difficult emotions and fears, and I appreciated Amy so much for that.

Still, I remembered Ashley's reaction when Dad threw the phone at her. The SMI could bring out a volatile temper that was completely uncharacteristic of the old him.

What would happen if he got out of control?

CHAPTER SIXTY-THREE

SENSE OF URGENCY

OCTOBER 18, 2022

"Wanted to let you both know," I texted Jackie and Keith, "that I just got a phone call. They are sending Dad to the hospital. His oxygen was low and he wasn't eating his food well. I'm going to call the hospital and keep you posted."

October 18, 2022
Amanda, 8:52 PM: His oxygen was at 82-84%. They're doing x-rays and told me to call back.

Amanda, 10:08 PM: He does have pneumonia. Weiss is admitting him. They have him on antibiotics, oxygen, and an IV. If he continues to have problems swallowing then he could end up in hospice but that's not a decision that's being made at this point.

Jackie: Hospice would be a bad thing—it means they'll make him comfortable until his imminent death. You scare me when you say that he could end up in hospice.

Amanda, 10:53 PM: Dr. said they're moving him to a regular room because he's stabilized. That's good for now. And they caught the pneumonia very early before he even had a fever

October 19, 2022
Amanda, 10:35 AM: They've put him on a smaller breathing mask device. Amy said he looked comfortable and says he feels okay (nods yes when she asks). They think he'll be there for a few days.

Amanda, 9:27 PM: I called and "talked" with Dad today. The nurse said he was listening and I believe he mumbled I love you when I said I love you.

October 20, 2022
Amanda, 1:09 PM: Doctor has Dad on the face mask oxygen, because when they tried to go down to the nose oxygen only, after a couple hours, his oxygen level dropped back to 81%. They want to see if Dad had a recent stroke, because of food aspiration, which they think caused this pneumonia. They can't do the MRI until they can get him off the face mask oxygen. The CT scan confirmed he had a large stroke but when compared to the CT results from last year, it's pretty much the same. He's getting IV fluids and they can't give him food yet so he doesn't aspirate until he's off the oxygen mask.

Amanda, 9:19 PM: They took a culture and they'll be able to tell within a few days if they're giving him the correct antibiotics for the pneumonia he has. I didn't know they could do that.

October 21, 2022
Amanda, 12:43 PM: He still needs the oxygen. Changing antibiotics because white blood count increased today, so previous med was not as effective as they had hoped. Trying to determine if it's the pneumonia still affecting oxygen saturation levels or something else. Running more tests.

Amanda, 1:09 PM: ruled out any major embolism in his lungs… could just be pneumonia… It took four phone calls, being on hold for eight minutes each time and getting hung up on at least once to get a nurse on the phone this morning. Probably short-staffed like everywhere else. Everyone I've talked to has been kind and helpful though.

October 22, 2022
Amanda, 9:34 AM: I'm going to vent for just a second… I have made over 10 phone calls between last night and this morning and, either no one answers the phone—it rings until the phone is disconnected—or, once I got the ER, they transferred me and then the line hung up. If I do get someone, no one can help me. "Please call back, the nurse is busy." Resident doctor has been paged to call me back.

Amanda, 2:55 PM: Dad is down to nose breathing tun whatever that's called, so that's really good. Probably means the new antibiotic is working. The thing they're waiting for is for him to be able to swallow again though. He's working with a speech therapist and they'll try again tomorrow

October 23, 2022
Amanda, 3:51 PM: Oxygen level stable on the nose tube high flow oxygen. He's not responsive to them other than when they ask "does this hurt?"

He still cannot or will not swallow food. Speech therapist will evaluate him again on the swallowing tomorrow.

Nurse said the next step if he can't eat would be an NG tube. That's a feeding tube that goes through your nose. I don't know if that's what Dad would want though.

I'm looking at the POA form he signed, and reaching out to Amy for clarification.

Amanda, 4:55 PM: On his Illinois DNR form, he specifically says do not intubate. Will speak with his doctor and nurse in the morning. And although Amy is out of town this week, she's having the owner of the company go visit Dad tomorrow afternoon and talk to the nurses. Will likely Facetime with me

October 24, 2022
Amanda, 8:24 AM PST: They are giving Dad nutrition through something called a TPN through an IV. This is not the same as a feeding tube. Waiting for the doctor to call me back. I need to understand if this is something they're trying to use permanently, or if this is a short-term solution

Amanda, 8:35 AM: Doctor phoned. They're not doing TPN yet. They're concerned about his CO2 levels, whether or not he's able to breathe that out sufficiently. Dad again did not pass the swallow test and cannot swallow water or food.

At this point, I phoned Keith and Jackie. Together, we reviewed Dad's forms and confirmed that Dad clearly checked the box that he does not want any medically administered means of nutrition. The air between us was heavy on that call. It's hard to comfort each other when we also need to be comforted.

The doctor said they would have to start TPN fluids ASAP. When Amy's boss FaceTimed me with Dad, I asked him to confirm that it was just temporary and through an IV line only. He nodded his head and agreed.

That afternoon, the doctor spoke to me separately. "I want you to understand that he can only be on the TPN fluids for ten days before we need to move to a feeding tube."

"You can't do that," I said. "That's not what Dad wants."

That's when I knew what I needed to do, not just as his legal POA but as his faithful daughter.

I needed to get to Chicago. Immediately.

PART FOUR

Understanding (2022)

CHAPTER SIXTY-FOUR

Dysphagia

OCTOBER 24, 2022

At the attending physician's request, I emailed them copies of his POA and DNR forms. I didn't realize that the only copy I had in my possession of Dad's DNR form was not signed by his doctor. His facility never forwarded the signed copy to me.

That hadn't been an issue until it was. I kept Keith and Jackie up-to-date with all news.

October 24, 2022
Amanda, 7:56 PM: Have a nonstop flight booked. I leave LAX tonight at 11:45 PM and get in at 5:30 AM to O'Hare. Rental car booked. Hotel less than ten minutes north of the hospital. Have to pack before I fall asleep from exhaustion. Maybe that's good… maybe I'll actually sleep on the plane.

Amanda, 10:10 PM: Never heard of this happening but the flight is scheduled to leave early because of some kind of planned power outage at LAX or something like that.

Who knows. I could get out there tomorrow and Jesus performs some miracle recovery and I fly back home the next day. And a giant asteroid could hit the earth… Anything is possible

Amanda, 10:29 PM: Upgraded to first class lie flat seats for an additional $299. I will accept that as my emotional support fee tonight.

Until the last second before takeoff, I spent every minute on the plane researching and loading information on my phone about dysphagia, the term I had only learned about in February. I searched for causes and treatments. I read then drifted off to sleep, worried about Dad.

The moment the plane touched down in the morning, I got in the car and headed straight for the hospital. I didn't want to get stuck in rush hour. I looked down and realized I was still wearing the same clothes as yesterday: my black work slacks and blouse. Who gives a shit.

I parked and rolled on another coat of deodorant then phoned the nurses. It wasn't yet 6:30 AM.

Fortunately, ever since Dad had been admitted to the hospital, I'd been such a pain in ass with my constant phone calls—but sweet as sugar when talking to anyone—that everyone on every shift pretty much knew who I was and a summary version of Dad's history.

"I read that the visitor's entrance doesn't open for several hours," I said.

"Oh, don't you worry," the nurse said. "When do you think you'll be here? We'll get you up here."

"I'm here now."

"Oh, you're in Chicago already? That's great. What time will you be here?"

"No, I mean I'm here. In your parking lot."

"Oh, wow. You came straight from the airport? Did you sleep?"

"A solid three hours. The turbulence was wonderfully helpful."

She paused. "Honey, come on up."

October 25, 2022

Amanda, 7:28 AM: They're giving Dad meds for pneumonia and he's still on the high-flow oxygen. Met with the resident doctor. We're going to have speech therapy here soon to do another swallow evaluation. I asked Dad about it and whether or not it's painful to swallow or the muscle wasn't working. He seemed to indicate the muscle wasn't working. But now he's under the impression that he can swallow and eat, but that's not reality. Just like when I told him he's getting medicine for pneumonia, he just said he didn't have pneumonia.

I snapped a dreadful picture of Dad hooked up to the thick oxygen tube, monitors, and IVs, hospital gown slipping off his shoulders and sent it to Jackie and Keith. I FaceTimed Jackie so she could say hi to Dad.

After I walked into the hallway to give her more medical updates, she got quiet.

"Amanda," she said. "I'm… I'm so sorry… but I can't… I can't come." Jackie sniffled and cried. "It's breaking my heart… to see him like that."

"I know he looks pretty bad," I said. I knew it hurt to see Dad like that; it hurt me, too.

"But if you tell me… if they say that he's not going to… to make it, or if you really need me there, I'll go… but I…I just—"

"Don't worry. I can handle it. If he gets worse and I think at any point that we're nearing the end, I'll let you know so you can be here."

And that's what we agreed to do. I understood that everyone has their emotional limit.

Prior to this, I never gave much of a thought about the importance of being able to swallow. I supposed I took it for granted that it was an effortless thing for most of us, a mundane but necessary task like breathing.

When Justin was a baby, he had constant ear infections. As a result, it affected his ability to learn how to pronounce certain letters and sounds. In elementary school, he met with a speech therapist who taught him how to fold his tongue or press it against his teeth to differentiate between the s's and f's and th's and other sounds to form letters and speak correctly.

I had no idea that a speech therapist also dealt with swallowing problems. Part of me hoped that, much like the speech therapist helped Justin overcome his speech issues, these professionals would help Dad overcome his inability to swallow.

CHAPTER SIXTY-FIVE

Reassurances

Dad kept screaming out to anyone who would listen: "I'm thirsty. I want water."

The nurses showed me how to use some spongy thing on the end of a lollipop stick to give him water. Kind of.

"You dip this into the water," a nurse explained. "And put it in his mouth. You can rub it inside his cheeks and he can suck on it. You can't do it more than a few times each hour or he could aspirate."

"But he's miserable." As soon as she left, I decided to cheat a little and sneak him more sponges of water when they weren't looking, as long as it didn't make him cough.

Dad became angry and at random intervals, he'd yell, "I want a burger! Where's my burger and pop? I'm hungry. I want a burger and pop."

What was up with his call for pop? Must be a Chicago thing. In California, we, including Dad, called it a soda.

Then Dad looked over at me with distant but pleading eyes and repeated his requests.

"Dad, trust me," I said. "I want nothing more than to give you a burger." His demands brought me to tears. I looked away so he wouldn't see.

I wiped my eyes and brought out my phone. I played Greek folk dance music for him.

"Do you remember all the times you took us Greek folk dancing?"

He nodded.

"How about this one?" I played Hava Nagila.

He shook his head. "Turn it off," he mumbled and closed his eyes.

"I'm sorry you're here," I said. "I'm sure it's scary."

He nodded, opened his eyes, and stared at my face.

"What are you scared of?"

He shrugged.

And so began a game of twenty questions until he conveyed two fears: one, that he wouldn't be able to eat; and two, that he was a bad father.

"Dad, that's not true. You were a great dad." I sat down by his side and took a deep breath. "If you weren't a wonderful dad, why would I be here right now? Why would I fly out from California to be by your side, to sit here all day and night?"

His blue eyes were moist at the corners and he stared at me.

"Do you know why? Because I love you. You were a great dad. And I love you, very, very much." I leaned against his chest and the cables and wires and tubes, and held my arms around him. "I love you." I couldn't say another word, because I had to concentrate hard not to sob into his shoulder.

From that point on, whenever his eyes opened, I pushed over my chair from the corner to his bed, and held his hand, or at least rested my hand on his.

The doctors started throwing out terms like LTAC, long-term acute care, and hospice, which apparently didn't mean he'd die tomorrow, but that he'd qualify for additional services.

Because, as I soon discovered, it was a teaching hospital, it began to feel like I was having to explain Dad's condition, medical history, and issues with swallowing to a revolving door of doctors and nurses. I quickly updated them on Dad's oxygen saturation levels and how many liters of oxygen he was on, and notifying them when he needed a new bag of IV fluids. Eventually they started asking me if I was a nurse.

The experienced respiratory therapist became my best buddy.

"The doctor said what?" He looked at Dad's chart. "She wants to bring him down to 20% on the oxygen."

"Is that a good thing?"

He shook his head. "With his numbers? No, he's not going down from thirty to twenty."

I didn't know what he meant but appreciated someone knowledgeable looking out for us.

I put in a call to Dad's primary doctor back at the nursing home, because I trusted him to answer the biggest question I had.

"How many days can he be on the TPN [total parenteral nutrition through IV]?" I asked.

"No more than seven to ten days," he replied. "He needs to be able to eat on his own by then, even if it's pureed food."

I wrote it in my notepad and traced until it was dark black: **Today is Day 2 on TPN.**

For most of the day, I sat on a chair in the corner and stayed out of the staff's way. I found that allowed me to stay past visiting hours. They had restrictive visiting hours, which didn't start until 11 AM, and didn't allow visitors to stay beyond one or two hours per day.

That was unacceptable. As long as I kept to myself, I became invisible, so they left me alone. Whenever they advised me that visiting hours were over and asked me to leave, I appealed to their sense of compassion by explaining that I was from California, my dad had been missing for ten years, and I needed to be by his side.

Getting up past security in the morning was an entirely different matter. I quickly learned the usefulness of saying that my dad was a "hospice" patient. That helped the most. Other times, the front desk had to call upstairs to get special permission. In those cases, I phoned them from the lobby to give them the heads up to help me out. I brought the staff cookies, too—thanks, Jackie, for teaching me that.

A hospital employee approached me. "The doctor would like your dad to move to Kindred, a LTAC, soon. There he'll be seen by specialists—"

"You mean not multiple teaching residents?" I asked.

She ignored my comment and continued. "Because he'll be stabilized from the acute condition he was admitted here for, the pneumonia. For the first couple days, he was hardly responding at all, so he's definitely improved."

"But what's going to happen after that? He only has eight days left on the TPN."

"He can get a g-line or a PICC line."

"You mean feeding tubes?"

"No, these do not go through his nose or mouth."

"It's still a feeding tube."

"This is not the same thing. He's getting TPN through an IV right now and—"

"This is temporary. What you're talking about is long-term. My dad does not want tube feeding."

"It's not technically tube feeding. They can also do the line which feeds through an IV into his arm or neck through his arteries to get to his stomach that way. So, it's not what it used to be. It's not a feeding tube."

Yeah, nice try. "Just because it's through IV tubing, that's dishonest not to call that tube feeding."

She sighed and came over to me and spoke in a sweet tone. "I hear you, but what does the family want?"

"What kind of question is that? My Dad is DNR and DNI. I'm his POA."

"I understand that. But have you talked to your family to see what they want to do?"

"I don't know why you're asking me this. It doesn't matter what the family wants. It only matters what Dad wants. Otherwise, what's the point of a POA document?"

"Honey, we hear everything around here. Families fighting. This one wants that, that one wants this."

"And so, people abdicate their POA duties? I guess you and I better have strong enough POAs to stand up to these stupid questions. And to answer yours, my sister, my brother, and I all want the same thing—for everyone here to respect our dad's wishes."

She shook her head and walked out.

What the fuck was that? I couldn't believe it. Is this how things really were in hospitals? Would someone designated to serve as a POA have to fight to do their legal duty? Unbelievable.

CHAPTER SIXTY-SIX

Perilous

WEDNESDAY, OCTOBER 26
Day 3 on TPN

At 1:35 PM, I parked the car near a restaurant to finally escape the hospital, get some comfort food, and decompress. I sunk my teeth into a massive juicy, crispy fried chicken sandwich. I'd never tasted anything so good. And I was acutely aware of every bite, every chew, every swallow with a newfound appreciation of what allowed me to enjoy this meal.

I ate half and packed the other half to take back to my hotel room mini-fridge, for two reasons: one, it would become my dinner in the lobby that night, and two, it was a break from the emotional stress. Before heading back to the hotel to drop it off, I sat back and listened to the rock music playing and closed my eyes, to focus on every note and lyric.

My phone rang. It was the hospital.

"Is this Joseph's daughter? This is the doctor at Weiss. Are you here?"

"I'm down the street getting lunch. Why?"

"We need to take your dad out for some tests, but he's refusing. He's confused and won't listen to us. We need you to come up here right away or they're not going to do the tests."

"I'll be right there."

Instead of getting up immediately, I paused for a few minutes to cry.

Thursday, October 27 - Day 4 on TPN

The tests showed that Dad's pneumonia was responding to the antibiotics. Beyond that, we still had the basic issue of him not being able to swallow food. He couldn't return home to his facility until he could eat, so we needed to find him another place with a higher level of care for him in the meantime.

I didn't know when I'd get back to California—I hoped by the end of the weekend—so I sent more lesson plans to my sub just in case.

After touring Kindred hospital, I sent them an email, because after what I'd experienced already, I wanted everything in writing:

> This is Joseph's daughter and power of attorney. It was great meeting both of you and speaking with you and touring the facility. I really appreciate the time you've both taken to answer questions. I feel very comfortable with having my dad at your hospital.
>
> To prepare for my dad's transfer from Weiss Hospital to Kindred on Montrose tonight, I want to make sure that Kindred hospital has my dad's DNR form and his POA forms on record so that his wishes are followed. Please include this information in his medical chart and forward it to anyone on his care team who needs to see it.
>
> You'll see from the forms that he has stated his preferences for quality of life over longevity. He's also stated he does not want any artificially administered forms of nutrition. He and I have authorized temporary TPN feeding through the IV and the midline, but anything beyond that has not and will not be approved.
>
> He will not be getting any G-line or PICC-lines or feeding tubes.
>
> He does not want any breathing tubes inserted.
>
> He has a DNR on record and his wishes need to be honored.

I look forward to him hopefully regaining the ability to swallow there at your facility through specialized testing like the x-ray swallow test and working with a speech therapist. This is especially important because we know he is already on day 4 of the TPN feeding today. We are aware that his doctor recommends 7 to 10 days, but that your facility may allow him to go up to 14 days through the midline he currently has.

We are hopeful that he will improve because over the last couple days he has been able to swallow 5-10 spoons of applesauce or pudding at a time, which is how he's been able to get his crushed medication including his psych meds for anxiety, depression, and the antipsychotic.

Do not discuss the mental health issues with my dad because he lacks insight, and if mentioned may make him upset and noncompliant with medications. Hopefully your psychiatrist will understand that and the need to maintain his medications.

After therapy and tests to regain the ability to swallow nutrition, my dad wishes to return to his home, the nursing home where he spent the last two and a half years.

I will be meeting my dad at your facility and as we discussed earlier, I would like to be able to be bedside with him throughout the entire day while I am still in Chicago before flying back to California.

Also, his family and I authorize you to share any medical information with and to communicate with Amy, the nurse the family has hired to help us coordinate my dad's care because all of his children and grandkids live out of state. My dad knows Amy well and I am cc'ing her on this email.

Amy responded to me right away. "That's great Amanda, keeps things clear. Let me know Saturday if you want me to come and see your dad while you're there."

"Yes, please, can you come? I need to talk to Dad about his options after day fourteen on the TPN fluids. I need you there. I can't have this conversation alone."

"I understand. I'll be there in the early afternoon."

I sat in the corner of Dad's room and snapped a picture of him asleep, his mouth open, and sent it to Jackie and Keith.

"This is how interactive he has been today," I texted at 10:21 AM. "But he was able to tolerate at least ten spoonsful of applesauce with crushed medicine, so that's good news. Doctor says Dad may be tired because he's back on the antipsychotics."

At 4:51 PM, I texted them again: "So this has been a super exciting day. 9 ½ hours after I got here this morning and I think I've heard four phrases out of him. But I need to stay here until 8:30 PM. They said that's when transport should be here to take Dad to Kindred."

By 9:44 PM, I texted: "Long ass day. Still waiting for transport. Should be a few more minutes, hopefully not much longer. Dad finally spoke to me fifteen minutes ago. He said he wants his hamburger and pop."

10:11 PM, with a few cussing emojis, I sent Jackie and Keith another message: "This is effing ridiculous. Original estimate: 8-8:30 PM I'm getting hangry." Then I added, "Although honestly, I ate half a small pizza at lunch, so, technically, I'm not calorie deficient" along with a picture of a new favorite food: Detroit-style burnt cheese crusted pizza.

A little while later, I gave one of my last updates: "Why is everything got to be drama around here? They finally got here and the nurse comes in and tells them that the other hospital won't take Dad if they get there past 11 PM. Nurses are quickly trying to get all the cords and lines disconnected while the EMTs are trying to get him moved over to the gurney at the same time. I'm checking traffic. It says it's a twelve-minute drive. It's now 10:45 PM."

I weaved through the city, alive with nightlife, crowds of young people meandering across the narrow streets. All I could think about was getting back to the hotel after Dad was settled in, and having a cold slice of pizza after midnight. Because, yeah, I was really focused on my health at the moment.

Friday, October 28 - Day 5 on TPN

Not surprisingly, I slept through my alarm, so I knew I'd missed the doctors doing their morning rounds. What could I do? I was only human.

I parked my car in the lot and crossed the street to the hospital, the one without an emergency room. Before heading inside, I answered a call from the hospice organization, who offered to help Dad with additional hospice care if we could get him back to his facility. They wanted to confirm our meeting in a couple hours.

"I'll see you then," I said. I watched a little girl, in a pink helmet, riding her bike across the street in the crosswalk. She looked to be ten years old.

Behind me I heard the sound of a car engine getting closer. Too fast. Too close. I turned my head to watch a huge black pickup truck barreling towards the red light at full speed.

I dropped my bag and shrieked. The girl looked up and swerved her bike just in time. The truck kept going.

My God. Life can be wiped out in a minute. And the truck never stopped.

Shaken, but relieved, I signed in at the front desk and headed to Dad's room. Quickly I realized that after dealing with screaming patients down the hallway, nurses liked to duck into my dad's room and told us how much they loved having us there, because we were so kind and didn't scream at them.

"A lot of patients do that to you?" I asked.

"Oh no," she said. "And sometimes it's family, not patients." And she went back out.

The new hospital was a huge step up. When he arrived the night before, they had cleaned him up. Today, they brushed his teeth, gave him lotion, and were extremely kind.

They didn't have Dad hooked up constantly to the pulse and oxygen monitors so there wasn't any more loud beeping like in the last place. They gave Dad lipids, in addition to amino acids, which he wasn't getting before. I felt more optimistic about the future.

The rep from hospice texted me that he was heading to our room from the lobby.

I counted out the days, and although it was day five on the TPN fluids, Dad hadn't eaten a full meal in twelve days, since he was admitted to the hospital for pneumonia.

It was at that moment that screeching fire alarms went off. I heard running down the hallways. The nurse popped her head into our room and said, "Keep this door shut."

Loud doors slammed shut in the hallway.

I glanced at Dad who met my gaze then closed his eyes.

Another text came through from the rep: Trapped behind a door... see you soon?

I opened the hospice brochures and kept reading while the fire alarm rang in the background and sirens rang out in the distance, getting louder.

False alarm. That's what they said. All of the fire doors reopened. Within minutes, the rep was there introducing himself to me and to Dad.

"He'll have additional medical staff coming out weekly, counseling visits, more people to keep him company, and I'm sure you read through our pamphlets for a complete list." He paused. "But you do understand, and so does he, that once he's enrolled in hospice, we in general will avoid sending him back out to the hospital. He'll instead be provided with comfort care where he's most comfortable, at the nursing home."

I signed the paperwork.

"We can't start his care here, but as soon as your dad returns to his nursing home, we'll schedule a team to come out and evaluate him, so he can qualify for additional services. From then on, our doctors and nurses will take over."

The speech therapist came by to re-evaluate Dad.

"It looks like he's following commands and swallowing okay," she said to me in the hallway. "So, I'll do the x-ray swallow test on Monday."

"What's that?" I asked. They hadn't done that at the last hospital.

"That will reveal whether or not there are hidden problems with possible aspiration pocketing or coating of the throat during the swallowing process. It that's the case, I'll have to put him on NBM status."

"On what?"

"Nothing by mouth."

"Then what if that happens?"

"I'll do five days of therapy and repeat the test the following Monday to see if there's any change."

"Then what if he doesn't pass?"

"The family should start having that conversation."

After lunch, I sat by his bed to hold his hand, but he pushed me away. He didn't want me to talk or hold his hand. He just wanted me to sit there on the folding chair next to him.

So that's what I did. And I debated what to say to Dad the next day when Amy got there.

I wondered if I should talk to Dad openly and honestly about what the test on Monday would determine and his options after that depending on the results. That way he could feel like he was more a part of the decision-making process. I also didn't want to upset him. But on the other hand, I also didn't want it to be a surprise after the fact.

Before I left that night, I leaned close to Dad and said, "I love you."

"I love you, too," he mumbled back.

Ultimately, Jackie, Keith, and I agreed: Dad deserves to know. If he's coherent enough, he should be involved in his own decisions.

CHAPTER SIXTY-SEVEN

MAKING PEACE

SATURDAY, OCTOBER 29, 12:30 PM

Before heading back to the hotel the previous night, I indulged in probably the best carrot cake I'd ever had with toasted pecans and freshly made pecan praline ice cream. Because why? I chose to eat my emotions that week.

Day 6 on TPN

I met Amy in the hallway and updated her on Dad's condition.

"So, basically," I said, "everything hinges on the x-ray swallow test on Monday."

"Does he know?" Amy asked.

"That's why I need you here. I don't know how to tell him."

"Come out with it. It's not easy for him or for you. If you need me to, I will help."

I held his hand and sat next to him on the bed. Amy sat on a chair on his other side.

First, I updated Dad on the family, because he wanted to know how Jackie was. I scrolled through pictures and showed him his nieces.

"Do you remember Keith, your son, Keith?"

He nodded.

"Do you want to know about Keith?"

"Yes," he said with some effort.

I took a slow breath. For years, I had avoided talking about Keith because of their estrangement.

This was harder than I thought it would be. "Well, your son Keith, after high school, he worked odd jobs, a movie theater, home furnishings store, and more, including Disneyland. But you wouldn't believe what he's been able to do since then." Dad's blue eyes were focused on my face. "Keith got a job as a bank teller and worked his way up. He was good at what he did and he worked hard." I took another breath, because I felt the weight of distance between Dad and my brother, and I knew Dad held regret. "Well, your son is now one of forty-some vice-presidents at the largest credit union in the state of California, one of the largest in the state." I continued lauding Keith's accomplishments, explaining some of the projects and positions he'd held along the way.

"Wow, Joseph," Amy said. "That's quite impressive."

"How do you feel? Are you proud of him?"

Dad blinked and nodded. And, with strained effort, he said, "I'm proud of him."

I bowed my head to hide my tears. But why should I be ashamed to feel? Dad needed to feel free to feel, too.

Amy and I explained the swallow test and dementia and how that contributed to the problems he'd been experiencing with swallowing food, and the aspiration pneumonia.

"So, ultimately, Joseph," Amy said. "We want this to be your decision."

"Would you rather them use a PICC line or G-tube or any other feeding tube if they determine that your body no longer allows you to swallow?"

He shook his head and closed his eyes and was quiet. I held my breath and waited.

Dad opened his light blue eyes, he looked from me to Amy back to me and said, "I want a cheeseburger and pop." Although hoarse and croaky, he spoke loud and clear.

"Now, Joseph," Amy said. "You understand the choice, right?"

"Dad," I said. "If you don't want the feeding tubes, then you leave this world on your own terms. Is that what you want?"

He nodded. "I want a cheeseburger."

"Well, goddamn it," I said. "Get the man a cheeseburger."

"I want to go back," he said. "I don't want to be here."

"I'll let them know." I stood up. "I'll go find a nurse."

After speaking with a couple of women at the nurse's station, I reiterated Dad's wishes. "He wants to return to his nursing home."

"The doctor will have to make that decision, and he's not going to do that until after the test results come back."

"When will he be here on Monday?"

"They're here early, around seven, make their rounds, and then they're gone."

"Well, I'm not waiting for Tuesday," I said. "I'll be here Monday morning."

I stood at the doorway to Dad's room and peered in. Amy was huddled close to Dad, talking to him. When she noticed me, she looked up.

"I need to get going, Joseph," she said. "I'll come back by the facility when you're back there, and I'll bring you a cheeseburger and pop. Do you want fries?"

"And fries," he said.

I waited in the hallway to speak with her.

"Amanda," she spoke softly. "You should know something. In there, I asked him if he was afraid of his enemies. And you know what?" She paused and stared into my eyes. "He said, 'no.' In the years I've known your father, he has never said he wasn't afraid of them hurting him or hurting you."

I smiled, tears in my eyes.

"You know why?" she said. "I think it's because you're here, by his side. He's finally at peace. Your presence has done that for him."

My shoulders shook with quiet sobs and she gave me an embrace.

"Stay strong. Have heart. You're doing the right thing. He knows what he wants."

Yes, he did.

Dad had made his decision.

CHAPTER SIXTY-EIGHT

Helpless

Dad chose a cheeseburger and coke and end of life versus tube feeding. Would I have done the same? Food brings me joy. Without family, without friends, without the capacity to move or eat, what joy was left? He wanted to leave with joy.

But maybe he didn't have to leave now. If he passed the swallow test on Monday, he'd have more time on this earth.

That afternoon, I showed Dad pictures of his family, but he preferred pictures of my dogs.

"Would you like to pet a dog?" I asked him.

He nodded. "Yes."

"Then when you go back home," I said, "I'll find a way to get a therapy dog to visit you."

He nodded then closed his eyes. I researched local therapy dog groups and bookmarked some pages. He drifted off to sleep.

When he awoke, I searched online for music. I played "Lighter Shade than Pale" by Procol Harum. When I was four years old, I remember sitting in the back of our maroon Lincoln boat of a car while my dad popped in an 8-track of the song.

"No," Dad said. "Turn it off."

So, I did. Instead, I tried Beethoven's "Fur Elise" and the "Moonlight Sonata," the two songs I knew he used to play and which I had struggled to learn on my own.

"Do you like that?" I asked.

He nodded.

"I have your piano books and your old piano at home."

He didn't respond but also didn't seem to mind as I let the song play out. Going forward, I'd stick to Classical music.

An hour later, a nurse entered, turned on a light, and moved Dad to change the fluid bag.

After she left the room, I asked Dad, "Do you want the light on or off?"

He didn't answer.

I repeated my question.

He yelled, "On!"

"Okay." I lowered my voice. "Do you want me to just sit next to you?" Every time, every day, since I'd gotten there, he'd nodded his head yes.

This time, he screamed, "No! Leave!"

What had I done to provoke his anger? I was here by his side for almost every waking hour for the past five days.

But how would I react to finally understanding the gravity of my situation? To be told my death may be imminent, all hinging on a single test. How would I feel? Furious, frightened, sad, filled with regret, or at peace? To know, to be aware that you can't remember things, that you can't swallow, that your body and mind are failing you… just because many other people had gone through it and would go through it in the future doesn't make reality any easier.

He needed some emotional space to process. This room, much larger than the last one, allowed me to slink back in a corner on the far end away from him. I kept silent, and because he was facing the window, he probably assumed I left.

I stretched. Maybe it was time for me to leave. It was nearly 5 PM.

A doctor stepped in the room and introduced himself. "Good evening, Joseph. I'm here to check on you. I need you to lift your left leg." Dad didn't budge. "Can you lift your right leg, even a little bit for me?" Dad didn't. "Can you raise either arm for me?" Dad didn't make a peep or even the slightest movement.

I motioned for the doctor to meet me in the hallway.

"I think your dad is confused," he said.

"No, he's not," I said. "He's being obstinate. I can see Dad understands you but he's choosing not to lift his arms or legs for you."

"Okay. So…" He looked down on some notes. "I see his central line came out."

"He never had a central line."

He looked at his notes. "Oh, wrong patient. Sorry about that. But he will be starting a g-tube on Monday."

"Absolutely not. He's DNI and DNR. I'm his POA. After Monday's test, he goes back to his nursing home, his home."

My God, I was exasperated. How many other families have the time to be by someone's side every minute to make sure this shit didn't happen?

Ultimately, I was so thankful I'd been in Chicago with Dad and that I'd talked to every doctor and nurse and therapist. I learned different medical professionals can be pushy with what they want to do with the patient even if it's against their wishes. And so many hadn't been able to "find" his DNR form that I now kept a copy in my purse and digitally on my phone.

It's incredibly helpful to have an advocate constantly asking questions and staying on top of every detail. It's too much for one person alone. It seems like very little info followed him from place to place. At Kindred, they only had Weiss records and couldn't access his nursing home records. I had to provide everyone with updates, especially the speech therapist who said the info was very helpful for her. I pushed to have tests done sooner, rather than whenever they got to it, prolonging his stay by taking their sweet time.

When I toured the hospice hospitals, I saw some very sick people hooked up to tubes and machines, and they were all alone, no family or friends by their side. Patients lie in beds, some with a TV providing background noise. It made me wonder if sometimes hospitals just keep some patients alive indefinitely to make money.

CHAPTER SIXTY-NINE

Homeward Bound

SUNDAY, OCTOBER 30
Day 7 on TPN

After dropping off half my lunch, instead of heading right back to Kindred, I instead drove to the lake. Dad loved Lake Michigan, like he loved Chicago.

Back in November 2004, when I toured through Chicago and New York with Dad, the wind was cold but the skies were a clear blue. Dad led me out to the end of the peninsula where Shedd's Aquarium was, not to go see fish, but to sit outside on the grass, surrounded by the lake.

"Look." He pointed to the skyscraper skyline. "You won't find a better view than this."

I ambled alongside a concrete walking path that edged the lake and leaned against the rail. Below me, water lapped at the rocks. The overcast sky with strands of clouds leading off into the distance, all reflected in the water. Yes, Dad, it is beautiful.

With my phone, I recorded the 180-degree view of the lake and stopped where the sky and water reached the shore.

When I returned to my dad's side, I held out my phone.

"Dad, do you want to see pictures of the lake?"

He nodded.

I turned up the volume so he could also hear the water hitting the rocks at the edge of the lake.

He nodded and closed his eyes.

I wanted to remind him of what brought him joy. Isn't that what we'd all want at the end? To remember what brought us joy?

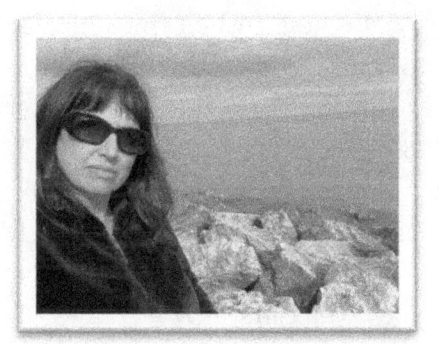

Monday, October 31 - Day 8 on TPN

6:59 AM. Despite my perennial existential crisis when it comes to waking up before the sun rises, it was worth getting to the hospital early. I was able to catch the doctor as he was making his rounds. He and I stepped into the hallway, out of Dad's earshot.

"Regardless of how the swallow test goes today," I said, "We want to get him back home to his facility. That's where he wants to be."

"Are you sure you and the family don't want to continue nutrition through a PICC line? It's minimally invasive."

"What the family wants is to honor Dad's wishes. He's DNR and DNI. He's clearly communicated that he does not want tube feeding of any kind, not through his nose, his arm, his stomach, none of that. He'd rather go to hospice. He wants a cheeseburger and pop."

"You understand that they may not allow that, there, either, if he can't swallow."

Who gave a shit what anyone allowed at that point, so long as he didn't choke to death or end up in pain. "I'll break it into little pieces. At this point, I want to give Dad what he wants." I'm sure I could get Amy or the staff to mush it up for him.

The doctor looked me in the eye and nodded. "Dementia patients prefer the familiar, so I can see why he wants to go back."

"Please, is there anything you can do to help us get him back there? I'm waiting to return home to California until he goes home."

"I'll talk with the social workers here and at his facility to get the transfer in motion."

Because I had learned how little information carries from one doctor or nurse to the next, and even from one day to the next, I told him I'd return by 7 AM the next day to confirm with him that the move would happen.

A couple hours later, when the speech therapist entered the room, my stomach balled up. This was it.

She unlocked Dad's bed and wheeled him out. "Come on," she said to me. "You can watch."

I followed her through the restricted doors with the Radiation x-ray warnings. I confirmed I was sure I wasn't pregnant and she handed me a heavy lead gown to put on.

"Just stay on the other side of the doorway." She lined up a series of cups and spoons and explained that each one had a different level of thickness. When she spooned something in his mouth, she turned on the x-ray machine and in real time, we watched the fluid go down his throat, pool in a pocket, and hopefully, after another swallow, exit down into his stomach.

When the food or beverage wasn't thick enough, it swirled in the throat pocket, but didn't go down.

"I need you to cough," she said to Dad and kept on him until he was able to cough enough to clear his throat. "See that? That means this isn't thick enough for him. That can lead to aspiration, gets into the lungs… then it can develop into pneumonia. That's what we need to avoid."

I swallowed hard, acutely aware of my saliva sliding down my throat. After watching her meticulously go one-by-one through the cups of varying thicknesses, I realized I would never think of swallowing food and drink the same. Seeing the mechanism, the necessary throat muscle movement, and the fact that your body can one day magically forget how to do it, I felt like I'd never stop worrying about choking.

"What was his baseline before the pneumonia?" she asked.

"I think honey-thickened liquids and mechanically separated food."

She shook her head. "Going forward, he is only cleared to have thickened liquid and puréed foods with supervision."

"So, he can eat again? Like yogurt, applesauce, cream of wheat—one of Dad's favorites."

"Yes." She smiled. "But not exactly what he was eating before."

"Dad, did you hear that?" I took off the gown and gave him a hug, which he seemed too weak to return. "We're going to get you back to your home by tomorrow. I can't wait to tell everyone the good news." I texted Jackie, Keith, Leo, and Amy—all were relieved. Dad was cleared to eat again.

I ran into the social worker in the hallway. "Do you know if there's anyone we can talk to, to try to expedite his move back there as early as possible in the morning?"

"The doctor cleared him to go back today. Ashley's working to get him a bed."

A bed? No. Not just any bed. Dad needed to be back in his room with his roommates, his space, his home.

"Ashley, please," I said over the phone. "He needs to go back to his room."

"We just moved someone in there today."

"But that's his spot."

"Technically, when he was moved from the hospital to Kindred, he was no longer our patient. But, since he's going into hospice, I'll see what I can do."

It took a village of people from both Kindred and the nursing home to get everything in motion to schedule Dad's physical move back. And the best part—he'd be back in his place in his bed closest to the hallway, in his room, back to where he felt at home.

CHAPTER SEVENTY

"I Love You"

When the ambulance transported Dad back into his room, his roommates welcomed him, as did his nurse Fred and Ashley. Fred hooked him up to an oxygen machine and put a nasal cannula on him. "Just for a little while, Mr. Joseph. Can I get you anything to eat or drink?"

Dad shook his head.

"It's late and it's been a long day," I said. "I'm sure he's exhausted. I'll see you tomorrow, Dad." I pulled up his blanket and gave him his teddy bear. "I love you."

"I love you, too," he croaked.

His roommate in the middle bed, nearest to Dad's, pulled aside the curtain. "You his daughter?" he asked.

"Yes." I went over and introduced myself.

"You're a good daughter. He's a lucky man. You're a lucky man, Joseph." Then he lay back down and pulled the curtain shut.

Tuesday, November 1 - Normal Food, Day 1

I slept well for the first time in a week. I packed up my bags—my flight would leave O'Hare at 7 PM—and drove to Dad's nursing home. Dad had a hospice evaluation appointment at 11AM and I wanted to visit with him before that.

Dad seemed more comfortable back in his home. The staff delivered his lunch.

"You want to help him?" the nurse asked. "He had breakfast, but I just didn't know if—"

"Yes, I'll take care of it." I showed Dad each item, but the first thing he wanted was his orange juice—he always loved orange juice. I peeled open the container of thickened juice and realized this needed to be eaten with a spoon.

So, I sat there, like I'd done when he was in the hospital before, and spoon fed him his juice, waiting every few bites to watch his neck to make sure he swallowed everything.

"More?" Dad asked after the last bit.

I went and asked for another one and fed him that and some other mystery meat and pureed food, it looked like jarred baby food, Stage 2. But at least he was eating, again!

"Next time Amy visits, I'll have her bring you a Big Mac and coke," I whispered.

He nodded.

Four people entered the room and introduced themselves as from hospice, did a medical exam, and asked him questions. They explained he'd need to requalify every six months, but that wouldn't be a problem, and explained the new services he'd be getting.

Then the nurse and aide left. The two administrators asked to speak to me privately downstairs to review paperwork.

We sat on the couches by the piano.

"When your dad goes into the active dying phase, we'll try to have him moved to a private room here, so the family can be with him," the woman said.

"How long does he have?" I asked.

"That's hard to say," the man said. "Every case is different."

"Yes, we've had some people in hospice for nearly two years."

"I hear what you're saying," I said, "but here's the reality: all three of his kids live in California. If his death were imminent, I'd need to know so that everyone could fly out here to say goodbye."

They looked at each other and he answered, "I'd say there's no rush. Although dementia is a progressive disease, he seems to be pretty stable right now."

"Dementia is a cruel disease," I said.

"We provide comfort medication and he'll be monitored."

"Can I show you something?" I took out my phone and found the video I'd recorded a couple days earlier while Dad was asleep. "Maybe it's nothing, but I noticed his breathing sounds strange."

I turned up the volume and hit play. It wasn't a long video, but when it finished, the two of them exchanged a long, but knowing, uncomfortable look.

The woman turned to me. "Maybe two or three months. Again, it's hard to tell."

"I'm returning in a week and a half with his oldest grandson. Maybe I can get an update from you then."

I returned to Dad's side and alternated between sending emails and playing games on my phone while he slept—still on a low level of oxygen through the nasal cannula—and sitting alongside him with my hand on his while he was alert. We kept going back to the orange juice.

"Dad, it's almost four o'clock. I need to get going. Got a seven o'clock flight. I'll be home before eleven, California time. Better to leave early to avoid rush hour traffic."

He nodded with his eyes closed.

"But remember, I'll be back on November 10. That's only nine days away, and Justin will be here, too." I stood up, gave Dad a long hug and a kiss on the cheek. I hovered over him and said, "I love you, Dad. I'll see you next week."

He didn't respond.

"I love you, Dad." I sat by his side. "Remember, Dad, I'm like you, very stubborn, and I'm not leaving until you say it back. I love you, Dad."

He took a deep breath, and with a hoarse voice, he mumbled, "I love you, Amanda."

Ha. I knew I'd win. I gave him another kiss on the cheek, tucked him in with the soft blanket Justin had chosen for him and the teddy bear with the Chicago t-shirt from David.

I got to the airport with plenty of time to spare and, although I couldn't usually sleep on the plane, exhaustion hit me and sleep overtook me.

Leo met me curbside and gave me a hug. "You look exhausted." He loaded my bag into the trunk.

I didn't say much on the way home and neither did he. And then my phone rang.

It was Chicago.

"Hello?" I answered.

"Amanda? This is Fred from the facility. I'm sorry to have to tell you, but..."

Dad had passed away.

I froze with the phone in my hand. Only hours ago, I was by his side. I was going to see him again in a couple weeks.

Leo turned to me. "What's wrong?"

"He's gone," I said with tears in my eyes.

Then I realized: Dad had waited for me to land safely.

I loved him and he loved me.

AFTERWORD

We made plans for Dad's funeral, a simple service. At that graveside ceremony, I FaceTimed Hilda who was stuck in Argentina thanks to a bad case of bronchitis; Jackie FaceTimed Keith who was on a European vacation. Jackie and I rotated the phones so that Hilda and Keith could say hello to each other before Laurie's husband recited the Mourner's Kaddish. Snow fell around us as we solemnly shoveled dirt over Dad's grave.

But that almost didn't happen.

Without a death certificate, there could be no burial. Without a doctor's signature, there could be no certificate. A week passed without either.

In death, as in life while he was homeless, Dad had slipped through the cracks—his fate suspended in limbo between a facility doctor who, after we signed hospice paperwork, was no longer his doctor and a hospice doctor who hadn't yet taken over Dad's care.

Humans are not infallible. Knowing this doesn't make it easier.

When loved ones have to face yet another wall, a little encouragement can go a long way and can come from unexpected places, like the uncomfortable middle seat of an airplane. En route to Chicago for Dad's funeral, I was nestled between two strangers, Robin and Wendy, who, after several glasses of wine and swapping of stories, offered selfies and support (we've since stayed in touch). Even a little moment of joy helps.

I had to fight it through to the end. It took patience and perseverance to bring Dad peace, but we made it happen.

On that cold November morning, the cemetery set up a tent for us to shelter under. Grass was still visible beneath the thin white powder. Laurie, her husband, and her mom were in attendance. Our new representatives from the trust company, Kevin and Alanna, were there to pay their respects. Jackie and Justin took a seat.

When the hearse arrived, the driver came around back, handed me the much-delayed death certificates and asked, "Where are the pallbearers?"

Pallbearers? We had none.

The driver pointed to every man in the vicinity.

Poor Kevin joined Justin, Laurie's husband, the hearse driver, and a cemetery employee in serving the role.

During Dad's short service, I read a poem for him and related memories of my childhood. "And I still love putting chocolate chips in my Cream of Wheat, because he always—"

"You did that, too?" Laurie interrupted me.

Chatter then laughter when we discovered that putting chocolate chip smiley faces in Cream of Wheat was a family tradition carried down from my father's grandma.

Laughter is good. So, it all worked out in the end.

Sometimes, even the strongest of us want to give up. Our hope dies. The world wears us down. We wave the white flag. But I didn't give up on finding Dad. I knew that finding him wouldn't cure him, but it would mean he wouldn't die on the streets alone. We achieved that and I told him I loved him. And if nothing else, is this not the ultimate success?

We had been gifted second chances: Jackie and I to tell Dad we loved him, Dad to tell Keith he was proud of him, Justin to see Grandpa again, David to meet Grandpa, Dad to be a grandpa and to express his love for us. Truly a dad to the end ... he made sure his little girl was home safely.

As I write this book, I'm reminded of the struggle so many others go through. There is complexity in human reactions. Our reactions affect others; their reactions impact us. But above all else, we are connected through our humanity. In that sense, you are not alone.

OBITUARY

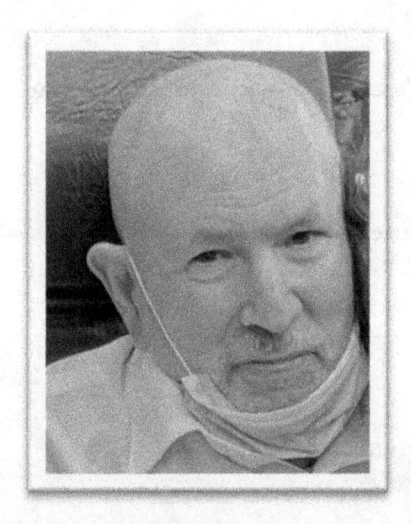

Joseph, age 79, of Chicago, IL passed away peacefully on Wednesday, November 2, 2022. Loving father of Jackie, Amanda, and Keith, and grandfather of four, Joseph was a kind man with a lighthearted sense of humor. Sharing the wonders of the world with his family and his love, Hilda, brought him joy. This included baseball, folk dancing, traveling, and exploring nature, both through hiking and photography. He was a quiet, gentle soul who will be dearly missed. His life touched more people than he will ever know.

RESOURCES

1. **LEAP Institute**
   Learn about Dr. Xavier Amador's LEAP Method for improving communication with family members who have anosognosia.
   www.LEAPinstitute.org

2. **National Alliance of Mental Illness (NAMI)**
   Find information about your local affiliate. They are an excellent resource for individuals and families affected by mental illness. The family-to-family educational program is outstanding.
   www.nami.org

3. **National Institute of Mental Health (NIMH)**
   Learn about mental disorders. www.nimh.nih.gov

4. **Treatment Advocacy Center (TAC)**
   Find information about the mental health laws in your state.
   www.tac.org

5. **California State Controller's Office**
   Search for your unclaimed property through the State Controller's Office: www.sco.ca.gov/search_upd.html (websites vary by state)
   In Illinois: https://icash.illinoistreasurer.gov

AUTHOR'S STATEMENT

Finding Dad, Paranoid Schizophrenia: An End to the Search is the follow up book to my previous book *Losing Dad, Paranoid Schizophrenia: A Family's Search for Hope* (10th Anniversary Edition). The first book, told through multiple perspectives, including Hilda, Amanda, Jackie, Keith, and Joseph himself, shows how a severe mental illness overtook my dad at the age of fifty-three. He had no prior symptoms, no drug or alcohol abuse, and no immediate family history. Xavier Amador, Ph.D., author of the book *I'm Not Sick, I Don't Need Help!* and founder of the LEAP Institute wrote the Foreword, which explains the neurological condition of anosognosia. *Losing Dad* is a fascinating story and I invite you to explore how everything in this book came to be.

Disclaimer: This book, *Finding Dad*, came about after extensive research and is supported through medical, financial, and legal records, as well other documentation including emails, videos, voicemails, and texts. Every effort has been made to insure the accuracy of the information in this text. Many of the actual names have been changed in order to protect the privacy of the individuals involved.

ACKNOWLEDGEMENTS

Thank you, Dad, for showing me on these pages how much love you had for us even though we didn't realize it. Thank you to Leo whose constant encouragement was the source of strength I needed to finish writing. I know I said the carrot cake I had in Chicago was the best ever, but you do make a delicious one, too. Thanks for sacrificing many board game nights for this book. Thank you to Mom for always believing in me—I'm glad you got to hold his book in your hands before leaving this world for the next. Thank you to Ken Elliott and Jenny Orci for your tireless help during the writing and revision process—you're both skilled writers whose opinions I hold in the highest regard. Thank you to Keith and Jackie; I couldn't ask for better siblings—we balance each other. Thanks for picking the perfect cover picture that encapsulates what we remember best about Dad: his love of nature. Thank you to Sierra, a talented photographer whose artistic eye reimagined the greenery. Thank you to William for answers to my endless questions. Thank you to Hilda who, despite the pain of the past, didn't disappear from our lives; I still want to see the penguins in Argentina with you. Thank you to Louis, Jill, Michelle, Dionne, Lilly, Nicole, and Lisa for your friendship and advice. A huge thank you to my editors: Jennifer Silva-Redmond and Laura Biagi. Your different perspectives on storytelling improved the crafting of my family's story. Thank you to Lynne Thies for your friendship and shoulder to lean on. I hope I have done justice to the family's story. And, once again, thank you to my readers. For those of you who are suffering: You are not alone.

READING DISCUSSION QUESTIONS

1. What is the theme of *Finding Dad*? In what ways can you relate to this story's message? How might the message be relevant today?

2. Grief is a normal part of life. Contrast how Jackie, Amanda, Keith, and Hilda processed grief differently. How do you deal with grief?

3. When a person deals with death, disease, substance abuse, disability, war, trauma, birth, job loss, financial loss, natural disasters, bullying, or harassment, what stages of grief are healthy, or unhealthy, for people to go through? When should someone seek help?

4. Sibling relationships can be complicated. How did the relationship between Jackie, Amanda, and Keith create tension or become a source of strength?

5. What are the signs of dementia and Alzheimer's? How did dementia and/or Alzheimer's complicate the treatment of Joseph's mental illness?

6. Do you know what options are available in your community for long-term care should you or a family member need it?

7. What are some examples in the book of expectations that were not in line with reality? Reflect on a time in your life when your reality did not meet your expectations.

8. Communication is important in a family. Think about the communication in your family. How well would your family be equipped to handle the onset of a severe mental illness or other tragedy or loss?

9. On average, one in five people are affected by mental illness, anxiety and depression the most common. If you are comfortable sharing, how has mental illness affected your life, if at all?

10. How do our mental health needs change as we age? How can we combat loneliness in our vulnerable older population?

11. People plan for the future with wills, trusts, advanced healthcare directives, medical and financial powers of attorney. But how prepared are you should your mental health decline? What about your spouse? Children? What legal forms are available for you to state your preferences for care should you be unable to do so?

12. How do you practice self-care?

ABOUT THE AUTHOR

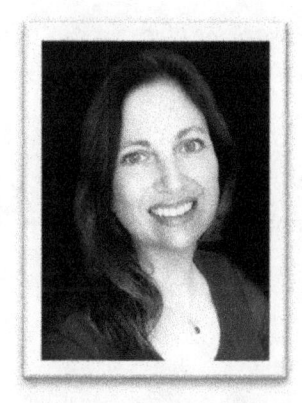

Amanda LaPera is national award-winning author. She has been a passionate advocate for individuals and families dealing with severe mental illness, due in part to her own family's experience. For ten years, she served on the Board of Directors for the National Alliance for Mental Illness, Orange County Affiliate (NAMI-OC). She resides in California where she enjoys spending time with her loved ones and furry friends. In addition to reading and writing, she finds joy in music, art, and nature, which she learned from her dad. Amanda is available for both in-person and virtual speaking engagements. Visit her website for more information: www.amandalapera.com

FB.com/amandalapera   Amanda LaPera   @desertstoryteller

OTHER BOOKS BY THE AUTHOR:

Losing Dad, Paranoid Schizophrenia: A Family's Search for Hope
(10th Anniversary Edition)

Look for *Desert of Dreams,* coming soon!